INTERMITTE]

EAT WHAT YOU LOVE, LOSE WEIGHT, INCREASE ENERGY AND HEAL YOUR BODY WITH THIS LIFESTYLE. INCLUDES DELICIOUS FAT BURNING RECIPES.

© Jaida Ellison

Legal & Disclaimer

The information contained in this book and its contents is not designed to replace or take the place of any form of medical or professional advice; and is not meant to replace the need for independent medical, financial, legal or other professional advice or services, as may be required. The content and information in this book have been provided for educational and entertainment purposes only.

The content and information contained in this book has been compiled from sources deemed reliable, and it is accurate to the best of the Author's knowledge, information and belief. However, the Author cannot guarantee its accuracy and validity and cannot be held liable for any errors and/or omissions. Further, changes are periodically made to this book as and when needed. Where appropriate and/or necessary, you must consult a professional (including but not limited to your doctor, attorney, financial advisor or such other professional advisor) before using any of the suggested remedies, techniques, or information in this book.

TABLE OF CONTENTS

INTRODUCTION

First of all, fasting is not starvation. Starvation is the involuntary abstinence from eating, forced upon a person by outside forces; this happens in times of war and famine when food is scarce. Fasting, on the other hand, is voluntary, deliberate, and controlled. Food is readily available but we choose not to eat it due to spiritual, health, or other reasons.

Fasting is as old as mankind, far older than any other forms of dieting. Ancient civilizations, like the Greeks, recognized that there was something intrinsically beneficial to periodic fasting. They were often called times of healing, cleansing, purification, or detoxification. Virtually every culture and religion on earth practices some sort of ritual fasting.

Before the advent of agriculture, humans never ate three meals a day plus snacking in between. We ate only when we found food, which could be hours or days apart. Hence, from an evolutionary standpoint, eating three meals a day is not a requirement for survival. Otherwise, we would not have survived as a species.

Fast forward to the 21st century, and we have all forgotten about this ancient practice. After all, fasting is really bad for business! Food manufacturers encourage us to eat multiple meals and snacks a day. Nutritional authorities warn that skipping a single meal will have dire health consequences. Over time, these messages have been well-drilled into our heads.

Fasting has no standard duration. It may be done for a few hours to many days to months on end. Intermittent fasting is an eating pattern where we cycle between fasting and regular eating. Shorter fasts of 16-20 hours are generally done more frequently, even daily. Longer fasts, typically 24-36 hours, are done 2-3 times per week. As it happens, we all fast daily for a period of 12 hours or so between dinner and breakfast.

Fasting has been done by millions and millions of people for thousands of years. Is it unhealthy? No. In fact, numerous studies have shown that it has enormous health benefits.

This has become an extremely popular topic in the science community due to all the potential benefits for fitness and health that are being discovered.

CHAPTER ONE: INTERMITTENT FASTING (IF)

Fasting, or periods of voluntary abstinence from food, has been practised throughout the world for ages. Intermittent fasting with the goal of improving health is relatively new. Intermittent fasting involves restricting intake of food for a set period of time and does not include any changes to the actual foods you are eating. Currently, the most common IF protocols are a daily 16 hour fast, and then fasting for a whole day, one or two days per week. Intermittent fasting could be considered a natural eating pattern that humans are built to implement, and it traces all the way back to our paleolithic hunter-gatherer ancestors. The current model of a planned program of intermittent fasting could potentially help improve many aspects of health, from body composition to longevity and aging. Although IF goes against the norms of our culture and common daily routine, the science may be pointing to a lower meal frequency and more time fasting as the optimal alternative to the normal breakfast, lunch, and dinner model. Here are two common myths that pertain to intermittent fasting.

COMPARING INTERMITTENT FASTING WITH DIET FADS

People experiencing intermittent fasting have proved that it does not cause starvation, tiredness, and other symptoms of daily dieting. It is because it is not the same as diet fads. It is completely different and has completely different results.

Everyone already knows dieting as a general way of losing fat. It is free of charge, simple and easy. However, the result it gives is not easy when compared to the hard work someone must go through while dieting. Sure, diets will help people lose weight, but it will not be a drastic change, and this change will probably take place after a few weeks of dieting. This is where the difference lies between diets and intermittent fasting. Following a flexible short-term fasting pattern will give an incredible result.

Not only will it reduce weight fast, but it will also show a drastic change in the body. This method affects the lifestyle of those doing the weight loss program. So, it can be a long lasting weight loss program. Another difference is that the phrase 'burn fat feed muscle' applies in intermittent fasting. Many people have proved while following this type of method that they did not lose any muscle mass.

HEALTH BENEFITS OF INTERMITTENT FASTING

1. Increases Metabolism, Leading To Weight And Body Fat Loss

Unlike a daily caloric reduction diet, intermittent fasting raises the metabolism. This makes sense from a survival standpoint. If we do not eat, the body uses stored energy as fuel so that we can stay alive to find another meal. Hormones allow the body to switch energy sources from food to body fat.

Studies demonstrate this phenomenon clearly. For example, four days of continuous fasting increased the Basal Metabolic Rate by 12%. Levels of the neurotransmitter norepinephrine, which prepares the body for action, increased by 117%. Fatty acids in the bloodstream increased over 370% as the body switched from burning food to burning stored fats.

2. No Loss In Muscle Mass

Unlike a constant calorie-restriction diet, intermittent fasting does not burn muscles as many have feared. In 2010, researchers looked at a group of subjects who underwent 70 days of alternate daily fasting (ate one day and fasted the next). Their muscle mass started off at 52.0 kg and ended at 51.9 kg. In other words, there was no loss of muscles but they did lose 11.4% of fat and saw major improvements in LDL cholesterol and triglyceride levels.

During fasting, the body naturally produces more human growth hormone to preserve lean muscles and bones. Muscle mass is generally preserved until body fat drops below 4%. Therefore, most people are not at risk of muscle-wasting when doing intermittent fasting.

3. Reverses insulin resistance, type 2 diabetes, and fatty liver

Type 2 diabetes is a condition whereby there is simply too much sugar in the body, to the point that the cells can no longer respond to insulin and take in any more glucose from the blood (insulin resistance), resulting in high blood sugar. Also the liver becomes loaded with fat as it tries to clear out the excess glucose by converting it to and storing it as fat.

Therefore, to reverse this condition, two things have to happen:

> First, stop putting more sugar into the body.
> Second, burn the remaining sugar off.

The best diet to achieve this is a low-carbohydrate, moderate-protein, and high-healthy fat diet also called the ketogenic diet. (Remember that carbohydrate raises blood sugar the most, protein to some degree, and fat the least.) That is why a low-carb diet will help reduce the burden of incoming glucose. For some people, this is already enough to reverse insulin resistance and type 2 diabetes. However, in more severe cases, diet alone is not sufficient.

What about exercise? Exercise will help burn off glucose in the skeletal muscles but not in all the tissues and organs, like the fatty liver. Clearly exercise is important, but to eliminate the excess glucose in the organs, there is the need to temporarily "starve" the cells.

Intermittent fasting can accomplish this. That is why, historically, people called fasting a cleanse or detox. It can be a very powerful tool to get rid of all the excesses. It is the fastest way to lower blood glucose and insulin levels and eventually reverse insulin resistance, type 2 diabetes, and fatty liver.

Taking insulin for type 2 diabetes does not address the root cause of the problem, which is excess sugar in the body. It is true that insulin will drive the glucose away from the blood, resulting in lower blood glucose, but where does the sugar go? The liver is just going to turn it all into fat; fat in the liver and fat in the abdomen. Patients who go on insulin often end up gaining more weight, which worsens their diabetes.

4. Enhances heart health

Over time, high blood glucose from type 2 diabetes can damage the blood vessels and nerves that control the heart. The longer one has diabetes, the higher the chances that heart disease will develop. By lowering blood sugar through intermittent fasting, the risk of cardiovascular disease and stroke is also reduced.

In addition, intermittent fasting has been shown to improve blood pressure, total and LDL (bad) cholesterol, blood triglycerides, and inflammatory markers associated with many chronic diseases.

5. Boosts Brain Power

Multiple studies demonstrated fasting has many neurologic benefits, including attention and focus, reaction time, immediate memory, cognition, and generation of new brain cells. Mice studies also showed that intermittent fasting reduces brain inflammation and prevents the symptoms of Alzheimer's.

6. Autophagy

Autophagy is the natural process by which our body removes out cellular junk to let new cell growth happen. It destroys parts of the cell, proteins and cell membranes which are not functioning properly.

How Autophagy Works

It is a biological process where the key players are tiny cells called lysosomes, which contain enzymes needed to digest and break down parts of the cell that no longer function properly.

That said, there is a dangerous side because lysosomes are very effective and a prolonged state of autophagy can lead to cell death; a process called autolysis. So a certain amount of autophagy is good, but too much can be damaging for our health.

Why this Cellular Junk Removal Process is so necessary?

Our body needs to regularly clean out any junk that is lying around in our cells, or else our cells become less efficient and deteriorate. When our cells are not working properly, our body becomes more susceptible to degeneration.

Autophagy makes our bodies more efficient, stops cancerous growth and metabolic dysfunction like diabetes and obesity.

How autophagy affects our cells

With it we keep our cells healthy. Our cells need cleaning from ineffective parts to avoid an imbalance between free radical damage and the antioxidants needed to prevent it. Without it, our body will experience inflammation caused by an oxidative stress. It is also necessary to keep muscle strength as you age. By removing cellular junk, your muscle stem cells continue to repair your tissues. This is the main reason detox is so important for older athletes.

CHAPTER TWO: INTERMITTENT FASTING GUIDE USING THE 16:8 FASTING METHOD

The 16:8 method of interval fasting is the most popular and simplest variant of intermittent fasting. Here you will learn everything about intermittent fasting 16/8, including instructions and important tips so you can start immediately.

Fasting has been an integral part of many world religions and cultures around the world for millennia. Nowadays, intermittent fasting is enjoying increasing popularity due to its many health benefits. There are several types of intermittent fasting. The method of intermittent fasting 16/8 is one of the most popular variations.

The 16/8 variant of intermittent fasting is a simple, convenient and sustainable way to lose weight and improve overall health enormously.

In this chapter, I'll give you an exact guide to intermittent fasting 16/8 and explain how it works and if it is right for you.

What is Intermittent Fasting 16/8?

The 16:8 method of intermittent fasting is simple and effective at the same time. Interval Fast 16/8 means limiting the consumption of food and caloric beverages to a fixed time window of eight hours a day, and dispensing with food for the remaining 16 hours. This fasting cycle can be repeated any number of times - from just once or twice a week to daily interval fasting.

With this method, your daily time window for taking meals is limited to 8 hours. The remaining 16 hours you fast and take no food. Within the 8-hour dining window, you can take 2-3 meals. This method is also known as **Leangains Protocol** and was known by fitness expert **Martin Berkhan**.

The 16/8 method of intermittent fasting is, in principle, quite simple, since your last meal of the day is dinner and you just skip breakfast the next morning. Interval fast 16/8 is a very popular form of fasting, especially if you want to lose weight fast and burn fat.

While other diets often set strict rules and waivers, 16/8 interval fasting is very easy to follow and can deliver impressive results with minimal effort. It is generally considered to be less restrictive and more flexible than many other diets and can be integrated into almost any lifestyle.

In addition to the positive effects on fat loss, 16/8 interval fasting also improves blood sugar levels and it has been proven that brain function and life expectancy are increased.

What Happens During Intermittent Fasting In The Body?

The intermittent fasting after the 16/8 variant is the trigger for a number of positive changes in your body – right down to the cellular level.

The insulin level decreases during your fasting interval, which improves insulin sensitivity. In addition, the blood sugar level is optimized and you turn yourself into a veritable fat burning engine.

A key advantage of short-term fasting is the persistent increase in human growth hormone (HGH), an important hormone involved in cell regeneration that maintains muscle mass during fasting and participates in the metabolism of body fat.

Short-term fasting also triggers important cellular repair processes in the body called autophagy. This ensures that waste and toxins are removed from the cells to keep the body healthy.

Other studies suggest that intermittent fasting is an effective defense against chronic disease and brain aging by making good changes to certain genes and molecules in your body.

Instructions For Interval Fasting 16/8

Interval fast 16/8 is easy, safe and without problems caused by needing to hold out for a long time. To start with intermittent fasting 16/8, first set an eight-hour window and limit your food intake to that amount of time.

I would recommend you to eat between 12.00 and 20.00. For many, it's the best time to eat at IF 16/8, as you'll be fasting overnight and just skip breakfast the next morning. For your first meal of the day, you will then lunch at 12.00 clock. So you do not eat and instead fast for 16 hours.

With a meal window from noon to 8pm, you can still have a well-balanced lunch and dinner and a few small afternoon snacks.

Example of a daily schedule and instructions for IF 16/8:

Your day starts at 7:00

Immediately after getting up your fat burning is highest

You skip breakfast - do not eat food - coffee is ok (no milk, no sugar)

In the morning you drink a lot of still water, coffee helps, if you feel a little hungry

At 12 o'clock you take your first meal of the day

No fast food or ready made pizza! Pay attention to a healthy meal (vegetables, salad, meat, fish, etc.)

In the afternoon you can have your second meal in the form of a small snack (a handful of nuts, hard-boiled eggs, yogurt, cereals, etc.)

At around 8:00 pm, you will have dinner and you will take your last meal of the day

After that, your 16 hour fast will start

The goal of IF is to keep your insulin levels low. Every time we eat food, insulin levels increase.

Milk in coffee, soda, sugary drinks, etc. All of this causes your insulin levels to rise and should be avoided during your 16-hour fasting phase!

When you first start interval fasting, your body is still used to having breakfast every morning. You'll probably always get hungry at the times you eat your breakfast. This is completely normal. Your body has "noticed" which food is fed at certain times.

Now that you know breakfast takes longer to appear, your body releases at the time of day at which you normally eat a breakfast that hunger hormone called ghrelin. But do not worry, that will lessen after a few days and before you know it, your body has adjusted and you will not be hungry in the morning.

I've been practicing interval fasting 16/8 in combination with a ketogenic diet for over 2 years now. And I actually do not feel hungry before 13-14, although I get up very early.

There are also people who prefer to eat between 9:00 and 17:00. At this time window you have time for a wholesome breakfast at 9:00 am, a normal lunch around noon and a light early dinner or snack around 4:00 pm before the 16 hour fasting phase begins.

Of course, you can experiment and choose the perfect time frame that best suits you and your everyday life. The important thing is that you are every day 16 hours fasting and eat no food in this time.

Regardless of when you eat your meals, it is recommended that you eat 2-3 small meals and snacks that are evenly distributed throughout the day. In this way, you can stabilize your blood sugar levels and control your hunger.

To maximize the health benefits of intermittent fasting, it is also important to keep your nutritious whole foods and sugar free drinks during your meal times. Eating fresh and nutrient-rich foods can help you improve your diet and enable the tremendous benefits of this diet with intermittent fasting.

Each meal should be combined with a good selection of healthy whole foods, such as:

- Fruit: apples, bananas, berries, oranges, peaches, pears, etc.

- Vegetables: broccoli, cauliflower, cucumbers, leafy vegetables, tomatoes, etc.
- Whole foods: quinoa, rice, oatmeal, barley, buckwheat, etc.
- Healthy fats : olive oil, avocados and coconut oil
- Protein sources: meat, poultry, fish, legumes, eggs, nuts, seeds, etc.

Non-calorific drinks such as water and unsweetened tea and coffee are allowed on interval fast 16/8. Even during fasting, these drinks can help to curb your appetite while improving hydration.

Unhealthy foods, lots of sugar and junk food can even negate the positive effects of intermittent fasting and end up doing more harm than good for your health.

Advantages Of The Intermittent Fasting 16/8 Method

The 16-8 intermittent fasting is a popular diet because it is easy to follow and flexible.

As a side benefit, you'll save even more time and money during fasting which you would otherwise spend every week cooking and preparing meals.

In terms of health, 16/8 fasting has a long list of unique benefits:

More Fat Loss: Restricting food intake to a few hours a day not only helps reduce calories throughout the day, but studies also show that fasting boosts metabolism and increases weight loss.

Improved glycemic control: Intermittent fasting has been found to lower insulin levels by up to 31% and blood sugar levels by 3-6%, potentially reducing the risk of diabetes.

Better brain function: Studies show that intermittent fasting can help to form new nerve cells to promote improved brain function.

Longer life expectancy: Although studies on humans are not yet sufficient, some animal studies have shown that intermittent fasting can extend lifespans.

Important Tips For 16-hour Fasting

Intermittent fasting is associated with many health benefits. However, it also has some disadvantages and may not be suitable for everyone.

Restricting food intake to just eight hours a day may cause some people to eat more than usual during mealtimes to make up for the hours of fasting. This can lead to weight gain, digestive problems and the establishment of unhealthy eating habits.

Intermittent fasting 16/8 can also cause short-term side effects such as hunger, depression, and fatigue. However, these "side effects" are short-lived and can be overcome after a few days, when you get into a routine and get used to the interval fasting.

In addition, some scientific evidence suggests that intermittent fasting may affect men and women differently, with animal testing demonstrating that it may affect fertility in women.

However, it has to be said that more human studies are needed to reliably assess the impact of intermittent fasting on reproductive health in women.

In any case, you should start gradually and consider consulting your doctor if you have any concerns or have negative symptoms.

Is intermittent fasting 16/8 suitable for me?

Intermittent fasting with the 16/8 method can be a sustainable, safe and easy way to improve your health.

Especially when short-term fasting is combined with an off-balance diet, a ketogenic nutritional plan and a healthy lifestyle.

Intervall fasting is not a diet! Rather, it is a way of eating nutrionally but should not be considered a substitute for a balanced and wholesome diet.

Although intermittent fasting is generally considered safe for most healthy adults, you should talk to your doctor before you start, especially if you have any health problems, prescriptions, diabetes, low blood pressure, or an earlier eating disorder.

Intermittent fasting is also not recommended for all women, especially when trying to get pregnant or for women who are pregnant or nursing.

If you are concerned about whether IF 16/8 is for you, or if you experience unwanted side effects while fasting, be sure to visit your family doctor.

Conclusion

During IF 16/8 you limit your food intake to an 8-hour window and for the remaining 16 hours you fast. It is very effective because it allows the body to reach the highest level of fat burning that occurs about 8-12 hours after eating a meal. In addition, intermittent fasting 16/8 supports weight loss, improves blood sugar levels, brain function and increases overall life expectancy.

Eat above all healthy foods during your 8-hour window and drink noncaloric beverages such as water or unsweetened tea and coffee (excluding milk and sugar).

If you have any health problems, it is always a good idea to talk to your doctor first before you start intermittent fasting.

Important FAQ'S: Intermittent Fasting 16:8

1.Where does the 16:8 interval fasting come from?

Phases of fasting are nothing new to our body. In ancient times, it was normal for our ancestors to have their stomachs empty for hours or days in times of scarcity. Once food was available, the reserves were replenished extensively.

As a rule, the body easily survives small starvation periods by storing energy reserves in various organs and tissues. If necessary, it can then fall back on this energy.

2.What must be taken care of during the 16:8 interval fasting?

It is important not to eat more in the phases of food intake than is usually consumed per meal. You should also pay attention to what you eat instead of indulging indiscriminately during the eight hours.

In addition, it is advisable to take only two meals and in between a break of 4 - 5 hours. If you take carbohydrates in between, no matter if they are biscuits, bread, dairy products or even fruit juices, then the body converts them into sugar. It goes directly into the blood. As a result the blood sugar level rises, insulin is released and the body stops fat loss. In addition, it may increasingly lead to food cravings.

3.No success in the 16:8 Interval fast: Why do not I take off weight with this?

If you do not lose weight despite the fasting phases, it may be because you just eat too much in the food phases. If you eat more than your body consumes, you lose the benefits of fasting.

Another reason may be the choice of food. Those who only eat unhealthy, high-calorie and sugary foods during the 8 hours can not hope for weight loss success. Only in connection with a healthy diet, the 16:8 fasting can lead to weight loss.

4.How much can you lose in 16:8 interval fasting?

Each body responds differently to a diet, and how much one ultimately decreases depends on different things. On the one hand, how overweight you were at the beginning of the fasting can make a difference, because the more body fat you have, the more the body can of course also break down.

On the other hand, weight loss depends on how you feed yourself and how much exercise you do during your time, for example.

5.Which drinks and food are particularly suitable for the 16:8 interval fasting?

Especially if you want to reduce your weight, the following foods and drinks are suitable:

- A lot of fresh fruits and vegetables
- Nuts and dried fruit as a snack, instead of biscuits and chips
- Protein and fiber-rich foods
- Silent waters
- Unsweetened teas
- Black, unsweetened coffee
- Superfoods such as chia seeds

6.Breakfast or dinner: which meal should be suspended?

The 16:8 interval fast is relatively well integrated into everyday life, no matter if you are an early riser or a night person. Lent extends over the night and part of the morning and evening.

If you are reluctant to have breakfast, the method will not be a problem and you can start with lunch as your first meal and then have time for a late dinner.

If you do not want to miss your breakfast, you can skip dinner and have your last meal in the afternoon.

Another option is to have breakfast late and have dinner early, for example, between 11:00 and 19:00.

7.In which pre-existing conditions one should not fast according to the 16:8 method?

- Do not use the IF 16:8 for the following pre-existing conditions:
- cardiovascular disorders
- chronic diseases
- metabolic diseases
- low blood pressure

Besides, not:

- during pregnancy and lactation
- with eating disorders or underweight

8.How do you do it in a safe way?

To follow the 16:8 diet safely, you must drink enough while you are not eating. Coffee or unsweetened green tea can be helpful (or pre-workout) the morning before exercise, as long as you do not use sweeteners or cream.

Consumption of a BCAA supplement is believed to prevent fasting muscle loss just prior to exercise. In the 8-hour meal period, it is essential to provide high-quality meals with all the necessary macronutrients, vitamins and minerals for the day.

Continue to drink enough and add enough protein to prevent loss of muscle mass. It can be hard to get enough calories in this short time, which can lead to weakness and dizziness.

In addition, you should be careful not to eat too much in your 8 hours just because there are 16 hours of fasting ahead of you. Intermittent fasting is designed to keep the body in a deficit for the day as a whole, so you should not over-feed high-calorie foods.

9.When is the best time to play sports?

Basically, the best time to do sports is the end of the Lenten window.

This way you can provide your body with all the valuable and important nutrients right in your food phase.

However, a sports unit should not be taken right after the last meal, as it may make you hungry in your next fasting phase.

CHAPTER THREE: OTHER TYPES OF INTERMITTENT FASTING

1. 24-HOUR FASTING

You don't have to fast for days or weeks to reap the benefits of this amazing weight loss and cleansing practice. Water and lemon juice fasting can do wonders for our digestion system and our entire body.

One easy way to get you started is trying the 24 hour fast! This is a great way to give fasting a try. It is also very beneficial to your overall health. Let's discuss this in more detail.

Fasting is done in two basic ways 1) Water Fasting and 2) Juice Fasting. Water fasting is recommended for experienced fasters only. Juice fasting is much more user-friendly and is very effective. People can fast anywhere from 1-30 days, although some people do go for longer. For most people, a 1-3 day fast is the best way to go and this will benefit you immensely.

Here Are The Guidelines

- **Hours of Fast** - I think the easiest is dinner to dinner so about 6PM-6PM. Why? Well, you are asleep part of the time, therefore your body is resting and you are not thinking about food. It seems to flow well with most peoples' schedules. Anytime is okay though, depending upon your schedule.

- **Before the Fast** - Eat lightly several hours before the fasting period. Don't stuff yourself with solid and heavy food. Eat healthy and light foods only.

- **Drink Juice** - Drink lots of juice. I favor non-pasteurized green juice and carrot/beet, but any vegetable combo is great. If it's difficult to find non-pasteurized juice at least buy organic/natural non-filtered juice. Lemon Juice with water (made from squeezing organic lemons) is another great way to help the body cleanse. And again some people use cranberry juice, but it needs to be pure juice, no sugar or concentrate. Any juice is good, but organic is best, natural only, and it should be only pure juice and water, with no other ingredients.

- **Drink Cleansing Tea** - Herbal & Green Teas help the process of cleansing your body. There are several fasting and detox teas, my favorites are made by Yogi Tea and Traditional Medicinals, or you can make your own. Cleansing teas and herbs are available at most natural food stores or online. Herbs are an essential way to help the fasting and cleanse process. Drink a few cups during your fast.

- **Drink Water** - Water will cleanse and filter out toxins. Drink lots of filtered water, which of course includes tea and juice. Pure filtered water is essential for your cleanse and overall health.

- **Eliminate Toxins** - Urinate and have bowel movements as much as you can. You will urinate frequently as you are drinking liquids. Tea and Raw juice, and in particular vegetable juices, will help you eliminate solid waste and cleanse your colon.

2. THE WARRIOR DIET

If you are one of those people who hate eating breakfast and find it much more convenient and enjoyable to eat one large meal rather than several small meals a day then you will not find the Warrior diet interesting but very enjoyable. The diet is based on the habits of ancient warriors who, in preparing for battle, ate little during the day but enjoyed a huge meal at night when they were less likely to be attacked and therefore could rest and enjoy their food.

Rather than a diet, it is a more an overall fitness program that combines diet, exercise and sound nutrition in a kind of feast or famine arrangement. The idea behind the diet is that during the day when you should be most active, you should eat very little. Eating a very small amount of food with no or limited protein stresses the body, making you burn calories faster, and adds to mental alertness. While this is only a theory many of you know from your own experience how you often feel sleepy shortly after eating, so the theory does make a lot of sense. By eating near to nothing your body and your mind are more alert because they aren't sated.

How Does It Work and Why Is It Beneficial?

This diet was devised by Ori Holmekler who suggests that it is not for bodybuilding, but instead for a way to develop a lean muscular body while at the same time keeping your size and weight down, in essence giving you a Bruce Lee look.

This diet works because of how your nervous system is set up to handle the digestion of food and funnelling of available energy. During the 20 hours that you are under eating, the Sympathetic Nervous System (SNS) is responsible for your ability to deal with stress, physical activity and periods of intense concentration. Basically anytime you need energy or cohesive body function it is the responsibility of the SNS to provide you with it. Whenever you eat, the SNS gets turned off as the parasympathetic nervous system (PNS) gets turned on, which is responsible for the digestion of food. This is why after having a big lunch it is common to have energy crashes and feel like taking a nap as opposed to carrying on with the day. Taking a nap anytime you eat a meal or a snack does sound nice, but who in this day and age has the time for that?

The overeating phase of the Warrior Diet will typically be during 4 hours of the evening. The PNS will be maximized during this time and will aid in resting, digestion and detoxification, among other things. All food groups will need to be consumed during this period of time; however, it does not mean that you should binge on junk food and sugary snacks. Usually, this will not be a problem because a person on this diet will crave the foods that the body actually needs as opposed to the foods that one might crave if they wanted to indulge their taste buds only. Of course, during the first few weeks or even months, there will be a transition period where you will need to condition yourself to lose the cravings for your old eating habits. This can be particularly difficult if you have a strong reliance on sugary foods and drinks. It has been said that a person's desire for food is the hardest to suppress, so this diet really does put this statement to the test.

3. ONE MEAL A DAY (OMAD)

OMAD stands for One Meal a Day; the idea is to fast for 23 hours straight and then consume one large meal in a 60-minute window.

Normally this involves waiting until dinner to break your OMAD fast, but ultimately it could be any meal with a 23:1 fast (it can technically be a 22:2 plan as well if you eat your one meal's worth of food slowly). People typically do OMAD to improve their health, lose weight, or both.

Because OMAD is a more advanced way to intermittent fast, it is a chance to get in on all the research-backed benefits like:

- Increased human growth hormone (HGH) levels, which allows us to actually build muscle and burn fat
- Lowered inflammation levels
- Decreased disease risks
- Increased autophagy pathways (cellular recycling and repair)

Another key benefit of fasting techniques like OMAD is that they enhance nutritional ketosis, which has its own anti-inflammatory, fat-burning, and autophagy benefits. Because OMAD is a longer fast, it tends to maximize these benefits. Longer fasting windows give the body longer periods of time to enhance all the benefits of fasting; breaking the fast earlier slows those mechanisms.

4. ALTERNATE DAY FASTING

This type of diet is based upon "calorie shifting" principles. Calorie shifting is a scientifically proven method of losing weight by eating more calories one day and fewer the next. The diets we will examine here follow these principles, but do so in different ways. The biggest advantage of eating this way is the effect it has on your metabolism. By making your body think it is not dieting, your metabolism will continue running high and your weight loss will happen faster and for longer periods.

Below Are Descriptions Of The Most Popular Alternative Day Fasting Diets:

- **QOD Diet**

The QOD Diet is a diet program based on a book that is all about on days and off days. On your "On Days" you are allowed to eat fairly regularly, but you must watch your sodium and potassium intake. On your "Off Days," you are relegated to eat only 500 calories and only 200 of them are allowed to come from protein. Again you are asked to limit sodium and potassium.

On top of that, you are asked to take supplements and protein powders to help regulate what you ingest. This will help facilitate faster weight loss according to the creators of this alternate day diet plan.

- **Up Day Down Day Diet**

This diet takes the QOD Diet a little farther because it does not require using so many supplements and potions to help with weight loss. It starts with the induction phase where you are on "Up Days and Down Days" (sounds familiar right?). During induction, you will be restricted to 500 calories and you are not as constrained by sodium and potassium. This makes the diet a little easier than the QOD. On down days you are allowed to eat regularly as long as you don't "purposely overeat"

That last statement is a little more ambiguous and tough when you are starving yourself the day before.

After the induction phase, you go to the maintenance phase where your down days are eating 50% of your normal eating routine.

- **The Every Other Day Diet (EODD)**

The EODD goes even further towards the ultimate alternate day diet. The EODD has different phases like the Up Day Down Day Diet, but they work the same in each phase. The reason this diet is more refined is that it incorporates the SNAPP Eating Plan which tells you exactly what to eat. So on "Burn" days, you eat exactly what the SNAPP Plan tells you.

On "Feed" days you can eat pizza, hamburgers etc. as long as it is during the times outlined in SNAPP. The rest of the meals you eat what's told in the plan.

5. FASTING MIMICKING DIET

Fast mimicking is a type of modified fasting. Instead of abstaining from food completely like a traditional fast, you still consume small amounts of food in a way that produces the therapeutic benefits of fasting.

A fast mimicking diet typically lasts about five days and follows a healthy protocol low in carbs, protein, and calories and high in fat. Calories are kept at around 40% of normal intake. This allows the body to stay nourished with nutrients and electrolytes will give you less stress than normal fasting but while still receiving the same benefits.

Long-term calorie restriction and long-term fasting can harmful, but fast mimicking is safer and more effective. Let's look at how much it differs from traditional fasting.

According to the advice of the World Health Organisation, consuming these five a day portions will assist any average person in reducing their risks of suffering heart disease, a stroke or a variety of cancers. The diet that includes these portions will also likely reduce the problems of diabetes and obesity, by helping to reduce artificial sugars in the diet and reducing our propensity in Western cultures to eat too much, which is what has led to the obesity epidemic all around us.

You eat 500-1000 calories a day for 2-5 days and on day 6 you return to a normal way of eating. It can be used for weight loss, fighting disease, and promoting longevity. Here's how it works:

> You eat about 500-1000 calories every day.
> Your daily macros are low protein, moderate carb, moderate fat.
> You eat things like a nutbar, a bowl of soup, and some crackers with a few olives or something.

Day One you eat about 1000 calories – 10% protein, 55% fat, and 35% carbs.

Day 2-5 you eat about 500-700 calories – 10% protein, 45% fat, 45% carbs.

Day 6 you transition back to a normal caloric intake with complex carbs, vegetables, and minimal meat, fish, and cheese.

6. PROTEIN SPARING MODIFIED FASTING

The idea of a PSMF is to reduce calories to the lowest possible threshold while still eating enough protein to preserve lean tissue mass and enough micronutrients to avoid deficiency. This is basically a kind of starvation, so you get the same metabolic benefits that you do with a "real" fast (which is also basically a kind of starvation), but the additional protein and nutrients make the whole project a little less risky and minimize muscle loss and potential nutrient deficiencies.

Practically, a PSMF involves:

Very few calories (typically under 1,000 per day – remember that the point is to induce a starvation response), with the vast majority coming from lean protein. Fat and carbs are minimized as much as possible.

A few non-starchy vegetables.

Supplemental vitamins, minerals, and salts to make up the inevitable nutrient and electrolyte deficiencies.

On a PSMF, the majority of calories entering your mouth are from protein, but the majority of calories you burn for energy come from fat; patients on a PSMF do go into ketosis. That's because you can't "burn" protein for energy the way you burn fat or carbs. The protein is just there to replenish muscle mass and prevent lean tissue loss – it's used as building blocks, not as fuel. Instead of burning that protein for fuel, you'll be burning your own body fat reserves so you essentially are "eating" fat – your own fat.

A PSMF consists of two phases. The first "intensive" phase lasts 4-6 months and involves severely limiting calories.

The second "refeeding" phase lasts 6-8 weeks, during which calories are gradually increased back to a more regular level.

7. FAT FASTING

A fat fast is a high-fat, low-calorie diet that typically lasts 2–5 days.

During this time it's recommended to eat 1,000–1,200 calories per day, 80–90% of which should come from fat.

Though not technically a fast, this approach mimics the biological effects of abstaining from food by putting your body into the biological state of ketosis.

In ketosis your body uses fat, rather than carbs, as its main energy source. During this process, your liver breaks down fatty acids into molecules called ketones, which can be used to fuel your body.

Ketosis occurs during times when glucose, your body's main source of energy, isn't available, such as during periods of starvation or when your carb intake is very low.

The time it takes to achieve ketosis can vary considerably, but if you're following a ketogenic diet you can typically expect to reach this state between days 2 and 6.

Fat fasting is designed to get you into ketosis quickly or to boost ketone levels if you have already achieved ketosis by restricting both your calorie and carb intake.

It's usually used by people on a ketogenic diet who want to break through an ongoing weight loss plateau or by those wanting to get back into ketosis after a cheat day, on which the rules of a low-carb diet are relaxed and you eat foods that are high in carbs.

A fat fast is very low in calories and high in fat. It's designed to create a calorie deficit, which is needed for weight loss, while quickly depleting your body's carb stores so you move into ketosis and burn more fat.

Thus if you adhere to this protocol strictly for 2–5 days, you may enter ketosis and begin burning fat as your primary source of fuel, particularly if you're already on a very-low-carb diet.

Nonetheless, a fat fast only last a few days, so large shifts on the scale can't be explained by fat loss alone.

The loss of your body's carb stores also leads to a loss of water, which is stored alongside glycogen, the stored form of glucose. This gives the illusion of fat loss.

8. BONE BROTH FASTING

A bone broth fast means you consume bone broth several times per day but not much other solid food. Fasts are not for everyone, and sometimes certain kinds can pose risks since they involve consuming little nutrients due to greatly reducing calorie intake. However, if you make a good candidate, consuming bone broth is ideal for a fast because it's chock-full of important macronutrients and micronutrients, including amino acids (which form proteins) like glycine, arginine and proline; vitamins and minerals; collagen; electrolytes; and even antioxidants like glucosamine.

Most people do best fasting for a period between three to four days, during this time consuming several quarts of bone broth daily and eliminating many problematic foods. One of the things that makes a bone broth fast stand apart from other types of fasts is that it's an ideal way to obtain more collagen, which is a type of protein needed to create healthy tissue found throughout the body. Collagen is found inside the lining of the digestive tract, within bones in bone marrow, in skin, and in the tissues that form joints, tendons, ligaments and cartilage.

Within collagen are other special nutrients, including amino acids like proline and glycine, plus gelatin which all have widespread benefits.

How To Start A Bone Broth Fast

Typically the fast lasts anywhere between 24 hours and 3 days, but we recommend starting small if you're new to fasting or consuming a diet high in processed food.

Most bone broth fasts consist of consuming between 3 to 4 quarts of bone broth per day while avoiding solid food and intense exercise. Fasting allows your body to burn fat, boost your metabolism, and heal conditions such as leaky gut due to its ability to restore good bacteria in the digestive tract. When you add in the numerous benefits of bone broth protein, the electrolyte and amino acid content hydrates, these come togeter to detox and heal your body.

Most fasting is done without solid food. However, if you are new to fasting or are feeling light-headed, it's okay to include one small meal of grass-fed meat and vegetables for every 24 hours of fasting.

9. DRY FASTING

Dry fasting is a type of fast that doesn't allow any water intake. The lack of water may help accelerate some of the protective effects you get on a regular water fast, like reduced inflammation and metabolic health.

However, it's a more advanced fasting method that only people who have previous experience with normal fasts should attempt.

Dry fasting has been perfected and practiced by many cultures and religions throughout history:

- Judaism (during Yom Kippur)
- Christianity (during Lent and Advent)
- Mormonism (one Sunday of each month)
- Buddhism (to aid meditation)
- Jainism (to reach transcendence)
- Islam (during Ramadan)

The Islamic, Mormon, and Jewish fasts are the only ones that prohibit water, so they're true dry fasts.

There Are Two Popular Types Of Dry Fasting Methods.

Hard and soft dry fasting is very popular. With the hard dry fast, the faster does not even allow water to touch their body. None!

When dry fasting the pores of the skin absorb water from contact with the environment.

This is one of the reasons many dry fasting experts believe it is best to practice in the outdoors, in the mountains as opposed to in cities.

This much cleaner environment is preferred as the skin absorbs water through the moisture in the air. Sleeping outside and near running water in this environment is ideal for longer dry fasting.

As you can imagine, the soft dry fast allows the participant to drink water during the fast. The presence of water lessens the beneficial and the uncomfortable effects of dry fasting but allows the faster to fast for longer periods of time. This is preferred for beginners.

10. JUICE FASTING

Juice fasting is a great way to get off the dieting rollercoaster and see real results quickly. Safe and effective when carried out correctly, juice fasting benefits your entire being.

Your physical wellbeing increases as the body is rid of toxins and excess fat.

Your mind benefits because fasting creates a stillness that brings mental clarity and helps you to develop will power and to better control your senses.

As you lose weight and feel much better about yourself, self-esteem improves and sets you on the road to what could be a life-changing experience, connecting you to your spirit and helping you to achieve balance in your life.

General Juicing Rules:

- Drink freshly prepared juice and do not store the juice for over 24 hours. If you can't drink it immediately, put it into a glass jar (filled to the top) and put a lid on it to prevent oxidation. Juice rapidly loses therapeutic and nutritional value during storage.
- Raw fruits and vegetables are not always compatible when eaten together. Apples are the exception. You can also mix pears with Jicama.
- Melons should be juiced by themselves. Making the entire meal melon is an option.
- Avoid using pre-bottled or sweetened juices. All the live enzymes are inactivated when they are pasteurized.
- Juices don't stimulate acids to be released from the stomach, but orange and tomato juice are high in acids

and you may want to mix these juices with other less acidic ones.

- Don't add more than 25% green juice to your vegetable juices. (Unless you have a barf bucket handy!)
- Juicing Greens--you might want to do this in between harder vegetables, as the juice sludges at the bottom and doesn't pour out easily if you juice them first.
- Dilute all fruit juice with water (one part juice to 2-4 parts water) and drink throughout the day. We've found that 2 cups fruit juice blended with ½ tray of ice cubes comes up to 4 cups--the perfect dilution and it's frothy cold.
- Vegetable juices need not be diluted.

11. TIME-RESTRICTED FEEDING

If you know anyone that has said they are doing intermittent fasting, odds are it is in the form of time-restricted feeding. This is a type of intermittent fasting that is used daily and it involves only consuming calories during a small portion of the day and fasting for the remainder.

Daily fasting intervals in time-restricted feeding may range from 12-20 hours, with the most common method being 16/8 (fasting for 16 hours, consuming calories for 8). For this protocol, the time of day is not important as long as you are fasting for a consecutive period of time and only eating in your allowed time period.

For example, on a 16/8 time-restricted feeding program one person may eat their first meal at 7AM and last meal at 3PM (fast from 3PM-7AM), while another person may eat their first meal at 1PM and last meal at 9PM (fast from 9PM-1PM).

This protocol is meant to be performed every day over long periods of time and is very flexible as long as you are staying within the fasting/eating window(s).

Time-restricted feeding is one of the easiest to follow methods of intermittent fasting. Using this along with your daily work and sleep schedule may help achieve optimal metabolic function. Time-restricted feeding is a great program to follow for weight loss and body composition improvements, as well as some other overall health benefits. The few human trials that were conducted noted significant reductions in weight, reductions in fasting blood glucose, and improvements in cholesterol with no changes in perceived tension, depression, anger, fatigue, or confusion. Some other preliminary results from animal studies showed time-restricted feeding to protect against obesity, high insulin levels, fatty liver disease, and inflammation.

The easy application and promising results of time-restricted feeding could possibly make it an excellent option for weight loss and chronic disease prevention/management. When implementing this protocol it may be good to begin with a lower fasting-to-eating ratio like 12/12 hours and eventually work your way up to 16/8 hours.

CHAPTER FOUR

COMMONLY ASKED QUESTIONS ABOUT INTERMITTENT FASTING AND SUPPLEMENTS

What is the most important supplement that I should be taking?

At bare minimum, everyone should be taking a multivitamin of some sort because of nutrient deficient soil.

I prefer organic, whole food vitamin sources such as powdered greens.

-What Supplements Should I Be Taking?

A multivitamin, an omega 3 source, a probiotic, and Vitamin D. As I said before, I prefer whole food sources over artificial multivitamins. So I would use a greens source as my multivitamin. I use a high-quality fish oil or krill oil for my omega 3 source. An alternative for vegans would be flaxseed oil or hemp oil. As for probiotics, the best source is naturally fermented foods such as miso soup, kimchi, natto, kefir, and sauerkraut. As for supplementation, get one that has more than 10 billion active probiotic strains per serving. Vitamin D supplementation is very important for people who don't get at least one hour of sunlight exposure per day. For instance, if you live in the northeast US, you will definitely need it. People with darker complexions will need more sun exposure than light-skinned folks because UV-B rays do not penetrate the skin as far. Therefore, less sunlight is converted to Vitamin D. The latest studies are saying that almost everyone is deficient in Vitamin D.

-What Is The Best Type Of Protein Powder To Buy?

It depends on what you are using it for. Whey is the best all-purpose protein. It absorbs fast, is cheap, and is best taken after a workout. Casein protein is best taken before bed because it is slowly absorbed. I would stick to a protein powder that is made from grass-fed cow's milk for higher quality.

-When Should I Take My Protein Supplement: Before Or After A Workout?

If you can afford it, both. The influx of branch chained amino acids taken before will give you a better performance throughout your workout. If you are trying to save money, the optimal time to take a protein supplement is within 30 minutes of completing your workout for recovery.

-I Have Tried All Diets And They Have Failed. What's The Easiest Way To See Results Without Dieting?

Intermittent fasting may work for you. Research shows that the 18th hour is the "golden hour". This is when you see the most results for the least amount of time. There are different theories on intermittent fasting. Some say the fast starts after your last meal and others say that it starts 2 or 3 hours after your last meal due to digestion. You do not want to fast over 24 hours straight. This is where negative effects on metabolism are seen and honestly, anything over 24 hours is miserable and uncomfortable.

-What am I allowed to eat during intermittent fasting?

Intermittent fasting is about not eating for a certain amount of time. There are no restrictions during the meal phase. That means all foods are allowed. There are no permanent prohibitions! And the amount or the number of calories is not limited in intermittent fasting. Even pure junk food consumers benefit from the daily meal breaks.

-Are medications and dietary supplements allowed for interval fasting?

Medication and nutritional supplements can be taken as usual during jntermittent fasting. Most supplements can even be taken during the fasting phase because they do not disturb the fasting process. The use of medication should not be changed on your own anyway, but only in consultation with a doctor.

Since intermittent fasting may decrease high blood pressure levels and improve insulin sensitivity of the cells, people who take medication for blood pressure or blood sugar should fast intermittently under close medical supervision. Here, if necessary, an adjustment of the drug dose is needed.

- Can I drink alcohol during intermittent fasting?

Alcohol provides calories and is therefore not allowed during fasting. In the dining window, however, you can also take alcoholic drinks. A general prohibition of alcohol does not exist in intermittent fasting.

-When is the best time for sports?

In principle, you can do sports while intermittent fasting at any time, both in the fasting and in the food phase. There are no concrete rules here. If you really want to burn fat, you should train on an empty stomach, because it promotes fat metabolism and afterburning.

-How long should I fast during intermittent fasting?

Intermittent fasting can be flexibly designed. You can fast every day for 14, 16, 18, 20 hours or more. In the classic variant, the IF 16/8, 16-hour fasting phases alternate with 8-hour meal windows.

How long your meal break should ideally be during intermittent fasting is not the same for all people. Again, there are differences that are partly due to your personal neurotransmitter dominance.

It's advisable you to start with the classic variant, ie IF 16/8, and stay for four weeks. This is the best way to find out if fasting 16 hours a day is too much or too little for you.

-Will I lose weight by intermittent fasting ?

How much you take off through interval fasting depends on various factors. Your current weight, how much overweight you are is just as important as the length of the meal break and of course, what you take during the meal phase to you.

There are numerous case reports of people who already lose weight with the IF 16/8 method without having to restrict their eating habits or count calories. Then again, there are people who have to fast for at least 18 or 20 hours without food and / or pay attention to their diet.

However, the fact is that intermittent fasting is definitely better for losing weight than traditional diets. That's because insulin levels are low for a long time due to interval fasting. This in turn is a prerequisite for the body to burn stored fat stores to energy and to keep the basal metabolic rate stable. So you lose fat faster than muscle during interval fasting, and you do not have to worry about the notorious yo-yo effect that calorie reduction diets trigger.

-How long can you interval fast?

With intermittent fasting, you do not have to do without anything permanently. There are no prohibitions. Favorite foods are still allowed. This and the flexible design of the meal breaks make intermittent fasting so incredibly attractive for long-term use.

Intermittent fasting is not a time-limited diet nor a temporary fad. This is the "original lifestyle" of man, according to his biological design and in accordance with the hormonal and neurobiological rhythms of the body standing.

Intermittent fasting is optimally suited as a permanent nutritional model in contrast to most diets. Short-term fasting can last your life - and with a clear conscience!

-Are exceptions allowed for intermittent fasting?

It may happen that invitations, parties or other occasions thwart your plans and you do not manage to keep the usual meal break. Of course this is not a broken leg. It's recommended simply making an exception and consciously enjoying it, rather than being a social outsider with astonished looks and tough discussions.

Nor is it a tragedy when 16 hours become only 14 or 12 hours. Maybe you just do not want to miss the breakfast with your loved ones at the weekend. All this is basically no problem. Practicing IF 16/8 5 or 6 days a week brings positive effects.

However, its recommened that you stay consistent for the first time of the changeover until you have become accustomed to the meal breaks. Otherwise there is a danger that you will not find the IF-rhythm after the exception.

-Can I continue the Intermittent fasting even when I am ill?

If you are ill because you have caught a cold or a flu, its better to listen to your feelings. If you are hungry, eat something, but do not force yourself to do anything. Often, when you're sick, you do not have an appetite anyway. In our eyes, this is a clear sign that the body does not need food, but puts all its forces into self-healing.

-Do I take enough nutrients with interval fasting?

Because you eat less often through interval fasting, some people are afraid that they will not get enough nutrients. However, intermittent fasting has a very positive effect on the gut. The long phases without food improve the intestinal flora and absorbed nutrients can be utilized much better again. There are no more effective measures than daily meal breaks to improve the nutritional supply!

-How often do you eat during the mealtime interval?

Basically, there is no rule for how often you should eat during interval fasting within your food window. So everyone can handle it the way they want.

People who eat small portions probably still need three meals on the 16/8 interval fasting method, which allows them to eat eight hours a day. Others, however, cope well with two large meals or a snack and a lavish main meal.

Regardless of how you decide to work it, from a physiological point of view you should not constantly snack during the food phase with intermittent fasting, but allow at least three to four hours pass between meals.

TWO COMMON MYTHS THAT PERTAIN TO INTERMITTENT FASTING

Myth 1 - You Must Eat 3 Meals Per Day: This "rule" that is common in Western society was not developed based on evidence for improved health, but was adopted as the common pattern for settlers and eventually became the norm. Not only is there a lack of scientific rationale in the 3 meal-a-day model, but recent studies may be showing less meals and more fasting to be optimal for human health. One study showed that one meal a day with the same amount of daily calories is better for weight loss and body composition than 3 meals per day. This finding is a basic concept that is extrapolated into intermittent fasting and those choosing to do IF may find it best to only eat 1-2 meals per day.

Myth 2 - You Need Breakfast, It's The Most Important Meal of The Day: Many false claims about the absolute need for a daily breakfast have been made. The most common claims being "breakfast increases your metabolism" and "breakfast decreases food intake later in the day". These claims have been refuted and studied over a 16 week period, with results showing that skipping breakfast did not decrease metabolism and it did not increase food intake at lunch and dinner. It is still possible to do intermittent fasting protocols while still eating breakfast, but some people find it easier to eat a late breakfast or skip it altogether and this common myth should not get in the way.

INTERMITTENT FASTING - HOW TO DO IT HEALTHILY AND SAFELY

Intermittent fasting can improve health, reduce the risk of serious illness, and promote longevity. Perhaps you're intrigued and would like to give it a go but aren't sure how to start. Or maybe you have tried it once or twice and found it too challenging. Here, I will give you strategies and guidelines to practice intermittent fasting safely and successfully. Please read the contraindications at the end of this chapter before doing a fast.

Intermittent fasting can be practised in the easiest way i.e 16:8 daily, meaning 16 hrs not eating and 8 hours eating. This can be done for a few months before starting another IF. A person may decide to eat 7am to 10pm (i.e 15 hours of eating and 9 hours not eating) and later move to 10 hours eating and 14 hours not eating and so on.

Follow the below guideline to effectively practice IF:

- Pick a day that isn't too hectic or demanding because you may experience some detox reactions. Make sure you have the option to relax if you need to. You will get more out of the experience if you make time to turn inward, still the mind, meditate, contemplate, and listen to your inner guidance.
- Enlist support from people close to you before you start. It's great to fast with your partner so you can both motivate each other and share experiences.
- Eat lightly the evening before by choosing a large salad or steamed vegetables with some lean protein. There is no point gorging the night before because it will make you feel even hungrier whilst you fast. It's best to avoid alcohol as well.

- Don't fight feeling hungry because you most probably will. Just be with the sensation without judgment, rather than resisting it (but read guideline 10 below).

- Engage in light exercise such as walking, stretching, and gentle yoga. This is not the day to do an intense gym workout or anything too vigorous.

- Add some breathing exercises such as yogic pranayama. A few minutes of practice offers amazing benefits from detoxification to boosting energy.

- Expect some detox symptoms such as headaches, feeling groggy, or short periods of feeling jittery. These are made worse if you usually have lots of caffeine and sugar in your diet. Avoid taking over-the-counter medication to reduce these side effects. Instead rest, go for a walk, and practice breathing exercises.

- Listen to your body's wisdom and if you feel unwell or it gets too much then have some food. Your body knows best.

- Break the fast gently the following morning. Have water or herb tea and a piece of fruit when you get up, then 30min later have your usual breakfast. Eat as usual for the rest of the day (you probably won't feel the need to overeat).

- During the fasting time, its much recommended to drink pure water or mix 1.5 litre pure water with a cup of black coffee or tea (no sugar, ofcourse).

Enjoy the changes in how you feel during and after the fast. Notice changes in your energy, emotions, and mental state. You may notice food is far more enjoyable on the day after the fast because your senses are heightened.

Recognise that it can take a few attempts to get used to this practice. After a few weeks your body will get used to it and the benefits you feel will increase as the discomfort simultaneously decreases.

Contra-Indications:

Avoid intermittent fasting if you are pregnant, diabetic, suffering from a serious illness, or taking any prescribed medications. If in doubt it is best to consult with your health care provider.

POTENTIAL RISK OF INTERMITTENT FASTING

The most common risk from intermittent fasting is dehydration. If you are consuming less then your body is taking on less water, it is very important you don't forget to drink on the days you do not eat. Water is essential and black coffee is often used if you get bored with plain water. With no food going in the stomach you are at risk of heartburn from stomach acid and long-term ulcers that can occur if stomach acid builds up against the stomach walls. The mental side of fasting also has to be considered. If you fast 2 days a week, don't over indulge on the other 5, keep to normal meals or it could lead someone to psychological disorders such as bulimia. You also need to be sure you are eating the right nutrients and minerals. Continue to eat fruit and vegetables. If you don't eat for 2 days, make sure the other 5 you are eating enough fruit and vegetables and not just binging or eating convenience foods.

PROVEN TIPS TO REDUCE HUNGER WHILE DOING INTERMITTENT FASTING

1. Balance Your Macronutrients (Protein, Carbs, and Fats)

Most people fail on intermittent fasting because they go very low carb and keep entering a state of ketosis which can be very detrimental for short-term bursts of high-intensity activity.

Carbohydrates: Minimum 0,6g per pound of body mass to stay out of ketosis.

Some individuals will also find higher carbohydrate intakes help them feel fuller.

It's better to keep fat between 25-30% of total calorie intake.

2. Don't Mistake Hunger for Dehydration

Hunger signals are often misleading – usually, we just need water.

To get an adequate amount of water carry a refillable bottle with you and aim for a gallon a day.

3. Tea and Coffee work wonders

Drinking coffee and tea is a great way to help curb your hunger while fasting. Before getting into the "HOW", first let's clarify what kinds of coffee and tea can be consumed without breaking a fast. When looking at coffee, any kind of BLACK coffee will not break your fast!

Black Coffee = No Creamers, Milk, or Sugar!

If you really don't like black coffee and need some sweetness in it, you can add any 0 CALORIE sweetener in small amounts, such as Stevia. When it comes to tea, the same rules apply; your tea must be BLACK in order for you to stay fasted!

It is also important to note that any HERBAL TEAS which include FRUIT are a NO GO while fasting! Fruit contains glucose which will definitely break your fast! Any black or green teas are good to go, also any spice based teas (ex. ginger) are safe as well.

How does coffee and tea curb your hunger? Caffeine naturally has the ability to make you feel satiated or "full" when consumed. It also helps with the mobilization of fatty acids in the body, meaning it helps move stored fatty acids into the mitochondria, turning it into energy, therefore giving you more energy. Having more energy will help you stay productive and distracted throughout your fast.

Green Tea: Let's take a quick look at green teas: Green tea can help decrease the hormone responsible for hunger in our bodies, called Ghrelin. When fasting, it's better you steep green tea in a water bottle overnight in the fridge. (Big Lean tip) When you wake up in the morning, drink the whole bottle before breaking your fast. This can help you feel more energized without feeling hungry throughout the morning.

4. Try Sugar-Free Diet Sodas, Flavored water (sugar free) and Sugarless gum

There's no evidence so far pointing that artificial sweeteners are bad for health so definitely give these a try if nothing else works and with moderation it should be fine.

5. Try a Tablespoon or Two of Psyllium Husk

Psyllium husk is a fiber supplement that helps massively with hunger, and it signals to your brain that you have food in your digestive system.

6. Brush Your Teeth

This has been proven to reduce the feeling of hunger.

7. Keep Yourself Active and Flowing

Do something you enjoy, and immerse yourself in activities especially during that morning period when you're most productive.

6-7 hours fly by very fast when you're in the state of flow.

If you don't have more work to do go for a short walk while listening to an audiobook.

By doing that you'll burn some extra fat, and learn more.

This is opposite of what most people are doing by putting themselves in a low consciousness zombie mode with TV and Social Media .

And we all know people eat because they're bored.

Stay busy, stay productive.

8. Get Enough Sleep

Shortened sleep time is associated with decreases in leptin and elevations in ghrelin which means more hunger.

A study comparing 2 groups that were on a 700 calorie daily deficit with 2 different sleep duration found that:

The 8.5 hour group lost about 50/50 fat and lean mass. The 5.5 hour group lost 20/80 fat and lean mass.

Research also found that:

"If you get 6 hours of sleep per night for two weeks straight, your mental and physical performance declines to the same level as if you had stayed awake for 48 hours straight."

As you can see sleep is absolutely critical not just for intermittent fasting but for everything in your life.

9. Drink tones of water!

The average person should be drinking around 2 LITERS of water a day, and most of us don't even get CLOSE to that! Drinking the right amount of water is super important for our bodies to function properly. When we are dehydrated, we can tend to feel low in energy, tired and HUNGRY. That's right! You have probably heard it before, but our bodies don't have "as clear" of a signal to tell us that we need more water (sometimes a headache), so instead, we feel HUNGRY, when really it is WATER that we need! Drinking tons of water during our fast can not only help us avoid feeling hungry, but it will also help keep us hydrated and feeling GOOD! During a fast, you have the opportunity to really monitor your water intake, making sure you are staying hydrated with the proper amount of water!

10. Carbonated water

Carbonated water can be a GREAT help when you are feeling hungry during a fast. Any plain carbonated water or 0 calorie sweetened carbonated waters are safe to drink while fasting (ex. Le Croix, Bubbly). Carbonated water can make you feel more full than regular water because it contains carbon dioxide! Carbon dioxide fills up your tummy super fast and can really help if you are having intense food cravings.

In conclusion, hunger during IF is only an issue for the first few weeks until your body gets used to the new schedule.

And the ideas I've outlined here will get you through those hard times. Now, most people are not hungry anymore 4-8 weeks into intermittent fasting. So it's safe to say that the hardest period is the first 2-3 weeks.

And to be fair if you don't notice improvements after 4 weeks then maybe IF isn't for you. Research scientists agree that it's not a universal must-do approach for everyone.

WHAT TO DRINK: PRACTISING INTERMITTENT FASTING FOR WEIGHTLOSS

1.Tea

If you are a tea lover, you will be happy to know that this hot drink goes hand in hand with the goals of intermittent fasting. Here are its benefits:

- **It helps reduce hunger**

It's a big point! When we do not eat as much as usual, we are hungry! This is due to an imbalance of the hormone of hunger, ghrelin. We must go back to this balance if we want to feel less hunger.

Catechins present in green tea, among others, have the effect of regulating the level of ghrelin in the body.

Otherwise, the amount of ghrelin will naturally decrease over time. The less you eat, the less ghrelin is produced.

- **It helps with weight loss**

Different teas can positively influence weight loss.

a) Catechins found in green tea burn visceral body fat, which happens to be the fat around the abdomen. Storing this type of fat can increase the risk of insulin resistance and type 2 diabetes.

b) Other studies have shown that white tea is just as effective as green tea in burning visceral fat.

c) The combination of catechins and caffeine in green and white teas helps to activate the metabolism, up to 4% in some cases. Having a good metabolism helps to burn more calories during the day.

2.Coffee

This contains caffeine, which increases alertness and helps curb appetite. Besides, caffeine also boosts metabolism and aids weight loss.

Therefore, drinking coffee is a great idea to control hunger and burn more fat while you are fasting.

3.Apple Cider Vinegar (ACV)

Apple cider vinegar contains mostly water and acids such as acetic acid and malic acid. 15 ml (one tablespoon) of apple cider vinegar contains approximately 3 calories. Perfect for weightloss!

WHAT TO DRINK: PRACTISING INTERMITTENT FASTING FOR AUTOPHAGY

Autophagy is a process of the human body that consists of destroying old damaged cells. If these cells remain in the body, they cause inflammation which then leads to other health problems.

The intermittent fasting already stimulates autophagy, helping to cleanse the body.

Green tea - contains active polyphenols such as epigallocatechin gallate (EGCG) as well as caffeine, all combined giving an extra boost to autophagy!

Bone Broth - Combining broth drinking with intermittent fasting leaves you with glowing skin, better hair and nails, reduced inflammation and a slowed aging process.

It doesn't matter if your goal is to lose weight or to generally improve your health – bone broth is a must in your diet.

WHO SHOULD NOT PRACTISE INTERMITTENT FASTING?

- Women who want to get pregnant, are pregnant, or are breastfeeding.
- Those who are malnourished or underweight.
- Children under 18 years of age and elders.
- Those who have gout.
- Those who have gastroesophageal reflux disease (GERD).
- Those who have eating disorders should first consult with their doctors.
- Those who are taking diabetic medications and insulin must first consult with their doctors as dosages will need to be reduced.
- Those who are taking medications should first consult with their doctors as the timing of medications may be affected.

- Those who feel very stressed or have cortisol issues should not fast because fasting is another stressor.
- Those who are training very hard most days of the week should not fast.

IF FOR WOMEN OVER 50 YEARS?

Obviously our bodies and our metabolism changes when we hit menopause. One of the biggest changes that women over 50 experience is that they have a slower metabolism and they start to put on weight. Fasting may be a good way to reverse and prevent this weight gain though. Studies have shown that this fasting pattern helps to regulate appetite and people who follow it regularly do not experience the same cravings that others do. If you're over 50 and trying to adjust to your slower metabolism, intermittent fasting can help you to avoid eating too much on a daily basis.

When you reach 50, your body also starts to develop some chronic diseases like high cholesterol and high blood pressure. Intermittent fasting has been shown to decrease both cholesterol and blood pressure, even without a great deal of weight loss. If you've started to notice your numbers rising at the doctor's office each year, you may be able to bring them back down with fasting, even without losing much weight.

Intermittent fasting may not be a great idea for every woman. Anyone with a specific health condition or who tends to be hypoglycemic should consult with a doctor. However, this new dietary trend has specific benefits for women who naturally store more fat in their bodies and may have trouble getting rid of these fat stores.

CHAPTER FIVE

HOW TO EXERCISE SAFELY DURING INTERMITTENT FASTING

The success of any weight loss or exercise program depends on how safe it is to sustain over time. If your ultimate goal is to decrease body fat and maintain your fitness level while doing IF, you need to stay in the safe zone. Here are some expert tips to help you do just that.

Eat a meal close to your moderate - to high-intensity workout

This is where meal timing comes into play. Khorana says that timing a meal close to a moderate- or high-intensity workout is key. This way your body has some glycogen stores to tap into to fuel your workout.

Stay hydrated

Sonpal says to remember fasting doesn't mean to remove water. In fact, he recommends that you drink more water while fasting.

Keep your electrolytes up

A good low-calorie hydration source, says Sonpal, is coconut water. "It replenishes electrolytes, is low in calories and tastes pretty good," he says. Gatorade and sports drinks are high in sugar, so avoid drinking too much of them.

Keep the intensity and duration fairly low

If you push yourself too hard and begin to feel dizzy or light-headed, take a break. Listening to your body is important.

Consider the type of fast

If you're doing a 24-hour intermittent fast, Lippin says you should stick to low-intensity workouts such as walking, restorative yoga, or gentle pilates. But if you're doing the 16:8 fast, much of the 16-hour fasting window is evening, sleep, and early in the day, so sticking to a certain type of exercise isn't as critical.

Listen to your body

The most important advice to heed when exercising during IF is to listen to your body. "If you start to feel weak or dizzy, chances are you're experiencing low blood sugar or are dehydrated," explains Amengual. If that's the case, she says to opt for a carbohydrate-electrolyte drink immediately and then follow up with a well-balanced meal.

While exercising and intermittent fasting may work for some people, others may not feel comfortable doing any form of exercise while fasting. Check with your doctor or healthcare provider before starting any nutrition or exercise program.

TRAIN YOUR BODY INTO A FAT-BURNING MACHINE

I advise that you do it gradually or you may be tempted to quit when your body is not given enough time to adjust. You will need to remove or reduce carbohydrate intake to the bare minimum in order to trigger this. Once your body has no glycogen to burn, it will tap into your fat storage to burn fat. This process is called ketogenesis. This process produces ketones into our blood, which are then used as energy.

Ketones produce much more powerful energy. They do not send our insulin level into a roller-coaster ride.

Some of the symptoms when you have entered into ketosis mode are:

- You will soon notice the difference when your body is adapted to fat burning mechanism
- You will notice a new-found energy that has not been activated for a very long time
- You will notice that your mind is clearer and has much better focus
- No mid-afternoon sleepiness

- You will be able to control your physical hunger.

I advise you to quit the following to ease the transition.

Sugar

The bad news just keeps on coming for people who love sugar in their diet. We are now aware of the difficulties that sugar can bring to our insulin levels, and with diabetes becoming more prevalent physical health issues caused by it are also becoming more common. Sugar can make food taste good and people can become addicted to it, but it is a product we would all do well to keep under 25 grams a day, and even less if we already have insulin issues.

But now sugar is becoming linked with mental health issues, particularly Alzheimer's disease and other dementia problems. These issues are becoming more and more evident in our society and once we have acquired these problems they are often difficult to control, much less eliminate. So what are the ways in which sugar, this poison that we put too much of in our system, can affect our mental health? In at least a couple of ways actually, and we will describe them here.

1. The brain and glucose. Some defenders of sugar have said that at least you need some glucose because that's what your brain runs on. Some experts are now under the belief that the brain fires on glucose only because

that is all that's available, and when it does we are finding that it damages the brain structure and function.

The really healthy fuels for the brain are other types of fuels, and particularly ketones, which the body produces when digesting healthy fats. In one test of healthy seniors who didn't suffer from any kind of dementia, higher levels of glucose were associated with poor memory, and the hippocampus structure of the brain was compromised. The shrinking of the hippocampus is considered a long-term precursor for Alzheimer's disease.

2. The liver and sugar, and what it all means for our brain. An essential building block for optimal brain function is cholesterol, which is produced in our liver. Our hard-working liver has many functions, and this is an important one, but also one of its critical functions is processing sugar. By increasing the task of processing fructose the liver has less time to produce what the brain really needs, which is that vital cholesterol.

We know that the brain has great adaptability, and by choosing a good diet, exercising regularly and opting for generally good lifestyle choices we can avoid many of the problems associated with old age. But in doing this we are pretty much on our own for maintaining the needed discipline. There is an entire industry promoting sugar and other processed foods, telling us that these dangerous toxic substances are actually good for us.

Other Dangers Include

- **Heart Threat** - Sugar has been shown to affect the involuntary muscle activity of the heart. A molecule found in ordinary table sugar called G6P has a negative impact on heart tissue at the cellular level.

Excess consumption of sugar and a sedentary lifestyle can increase a person's risk of developing heart failure. Heart failure often claims peoples lives in less than a decade after diagnosis.

- **Belly Fat** - There has been an alarming rise in obesity rates in teenagers and small children over these past few decades. One of the major contributing factors to this trend is an increase in the consumption of fructose. Fructose is an inexpensive form of sugar used in soda, ice cream, cookies and even bread products.

Fructose appears to boost the growth of visceral fat or the fat found in our midsections. When a child develops mature visceral fat early in life, he/she has a higher risk of being obese in adulthood.

- **Deadly Appetite** - Our bodies are naturally equipped with mechanisms that tell us when to stop eating. Studies show that sugar has found a way to suspend those natural mechanisms. Consuming foods and beverages rich in sugar contributes to the development of a condition called leptin resistance.

When a person has leptin resistance they don't feel full and satisfied with moderate amounts of food, so they continue consuming excessive amounts of food every time they eat.

Our bodies also have a tough time detecting the presence of sugar in beverages. It's difficult for the body to send a signal that you already consumed a lot of calories from soda or juices because this substance just doesn't register the same way as other types of food.

- Reduces our natural defense against bacterial defense (infectious disease)
- Leads to cancer
- Weakens eyesight
- Causes hypoglycemia and diabetes
- Causes a rapid adrenaline levels rise in children
- Causes premature aging
- Contributes to obesity
- Increases the risk of Crohn's disease
- Causes arthritis
- Causes asthma
- Causes gallstones
- Causes heart disease
- Causes hemorrhoids

- Causes varicose veins
- Decreases growth hormones
- Increases cholesterol
- Interferes with the absorption of protein
- Causes food allergies
- Causes cataracts
- Ages our skin
- Increases the size of our liver and kidneys
- Makes tendons more brittle
- Causes headaches and migraines
- Increases the risk of getting gout
- Can contribute to Alzheimer's disease
- Causes dizziness
- Is addictive

Withdrawal effects of quitting sugar

It took me about a year to consciously remove sugar from my diet. Once you have gone through that, you will live with so much energy without craving sugary food.

When you significantly slash your sugar intake, it can cause your blood sugar to drop, which can result in a host of symptoms as your body starts to adapt to finding new sources of energy. Sugar withdrawal nausea, headaches and fatigue are just a few of the typical side effects many report as a result of sugar withdrawal.

Of course, the severity of your symptoms largely depends on the amount of sugar in your diet beforehand. If you were loading up on the candy and sweet treats before, you're more likely to experience some of these symptoms than if sugar made up only a small part of your diet previously.

Some Of The Most Common Symptoms Caused By Sugar Withdrawal Include:

- Headaches
- Bloating
- Nausea
- Muscle aches
- Diarrhea
- Fatigue
- Hunger
- Anxiety
- Depression
- Cravings
- Chills

SUGAR WITHDRAWAL STAGES

Although the list of common side effects can be a bit daunting, keep in mind that these symptoms are temporary and generally only last a few days for most people. Here are the stages you can expect to encounter when you decide to drop sugar from your diet:

1. Feeling Motivated

When you make the decision to kick sugar to the curb, you will likely feel highly motivated and ready to reap the rewards of a healthier diet and lifestyle. Keep it up, as you'll need this motivation to propel you through the cravings, headaches and fatigue yet to come.

2. Cravings Start to Kick In

Cravings are one of the earliest signs of sugar withdrawal. Many people, for instance, establish a routine with their diets, and may find themselves glancing over at the vending machine when that mid-morning hunger starts to set in.

During this phase it's best to prepare by keeping healthy snacks at hand so it's even easier to resist the urge to indulge in your favorite sweets.

3. Symptoms Peak

Soon after the cravings hit, you may begin to experience some of the previously mentioned sugar withdrawal symptoms. Headaches, hunger, chills and even sugar withdrawal diarrhea can set in and make it harder than ever to stay motivated.

Remember why you decided to start eating more healthily and use that to keep you driven and determined to stay on the path to better health.

4. You Start to Feel Better

Once your symptoms start to clear up, you'll likely find yourself feeling better than ever. Many people have reported improvements in skin health, reduced brain fog and a boost in energy levels as a result of giving up added sugar.

Plus, by following a healthy diet and including more nutrient-dense foods in your day, you'll enjoy a lower risk of chronic disease and better overall health as well.

HOW TO REDUCE SUGAR CRAVINGS

First of all, do not try to cut yourself off from sugar altogether. While it may be tempting to cut it all out at once, this is a sure recipe for giving up and relapsing. Instead, try cutting one or two sugary foods out of your diet at a time. If you love soda, cookies, and a nightly bowl of ice cream, choose one of these at a time and find a healthier replacement. Instead of soda, try drinking fruit tea or water with a splash of fruit juice. If you love cookies, try making them yourself or eating fruit instead. If you wonder what you would do without your nightly bowl of ice cream, try a small square of organic dark chocolate instead. With substitutions like these, you will find it easier and easier to manage your sugar cravings without turning to processed sweets.

Once you've started controlling or eliminating the obvious sugars in your diet, start looking for the hidden sugars that you don't realize you are consuming. Make a habit of reading the label of everything that you purchase. You will be surprised at how many foods contain sugar or corn syrup as ingredients, even if they are not naturally sweet.

Making a conscious choice to purchase foods without added sugars is an excellent way to conquer your sugar cravings and reduce the amount of sugar that you are consuming.

If you still find yourself craving sugar, the next thing to try is a distraction. Strenuous exercise will help to distract you from your sugar cravings. As an added bonus exercise releases endorphins, which mimic the "high" that you get from eating sugary food but in a healthy way. Besides this, most people are reluctant to counteract the calorie burning effects of a strenuous workout with a pint of high fat ice cream.

Lastly, remember to give yourself a break. Allow yourself one healthy sweet per day. This could be a square of organic dark chocolate, a small bowl of natural ice cream, or even a piece of fruit that you've been saving. Reminding yourself that you have a treat waiting at home is an excellent way to motivate yourself to resist the sugar cravings that plague you as you are going through your daily routine.

DIFFERENT CHEMICAL ALTERNATIVE NAMES OF SUGAR

Sugar smells sweet and tastes sweet, but what about its name? How many sugar names are there? How many definitions? We use sugar to mean so many things, and food manufacturers often use it to disguise how bad the food is that we are eating.

"What's in a name? That which we call a rose by any other name would smell as sweet."

Added sugar goes by many names, and most types consist of glucose and/or fructose. High-fructose added sugars are more harmful.

1. Sugar/Sucrose

Sucrose is the most common type of sugar.

Often called "table sugar," it is a naturally occurring carbohydrate found in many fruits and plants.

Table sugar is usually extracted from sugar cane or sugar beets. It consists of 50% glucose and 50% fructose, bound together.

Sucrose is found in many foods, including ice cream, candy, pastries, cookies, soda, fruit juices, canned fruit, processed meat, breakfast cereals and ketchup, to name a few.

2. High-Fructose Corn Syrup (HFCS)

High-fructose corn syrup is a widely used sweetener, especially in the US.

It is produced from corn starch via an industrial process and consists of both fructose and glucose.

There are several different types of HFCS, which contain varying amounts of fructose.

Two notable varieties are:

- HFCS 55: This is the most common type of HFCS. It contains 55% fructose and 45% glucose, which makes it similar to sucrose in composition.
- HFCS 90: This form contains 90% fructose.

High-fructose corn syrup is found in many foods, especially in the US. These include soda, breads, cookies, candy, ice cream, cakes, cereal bars and many others.

3. Agave Nectar

Agave nectar, also called agave syrup, is a very popular sweetener produced from the agave plant.

It is commonly used as a "healthy" alternative to sugar because it doesn't spike blood sugar levels as much as many other sugar varieties.

However, agave nectar contains about 70–90% fructose, and 10–30% glucose.

Given the harmful health effects of excess fructose consumption, agave nectar may be even worse for metabolic health than regular sugar.

It is used in many "health foods," such as fruit bars, sweetened yogurts and cereal bars.

4-37. Other Sugars With Glucose and Fructose

Most added sugars and sweeteners contain both glucose and fructose.

Here are a few examples:

- Beet sugar
- Blackstrap molasses
- Brown sugar
- Buttered syrup
- Cane juice crystals
- Cane sugar
- Caramel
- Carob syrup
- Castor sugar
- Coconut sugar
- Confectioner's sugar (powdered sugar)

- Date sugar
- Demerara sugar
- Evaporated cane juice
- Florida Crystals
- Fruit juice
- Fruit juice concentrate
- Golden sugar
- Golden syrup
- Grape sugar
- Honey
- Icing sugar
- Invert sugar
- Maple syrup
- Molasses
- Muscovado sugar
- Panela sugar
- Raw sugar
- Refiner's syrup
- Sorghum syrup
- Sucanat
- Treacle sugar
- Turbinado sugar
- Yellow sugar

38–52. Sugars With Glucose

These sweeteners contain glucose, either pure or combined with sugars other than fructose (such as other glucose units or galactose):

- Barley malt
- Brown rice syrup
- Corn syrup
- Corn syrup solids
- Dextrin
- Dextrose
- Diastatic malt
- Ethyl maltol
- Glucose
- Glucose solids
- Lactose
- Malt syrup
- Maltodextrin
- Maltose
- Rice syrup

53–54. Sugars With Fructose Only

These two sweeteners contain only fructose:

- Crystalline fructose
- Fructose

55–56. Other Sugars

There are a few added sugars that contain neither glucose nor fructose. They are less sweet and less common, but are sometimes used as sweeteners:

- D-ribose
- Galactose

There was nothing that i enjoyed much more than sipping a cup of Earl Grey with a spoonful of sugar. I used to drink that every weekend. I had to quit doing that considering the harm it did to my body. At this moment, I have no slight craving to drink tea (with sugar) anymore, and when a certain food contains a little sugar, I would be able to taste the sweetness when others may not taste the sweetness.

As parents of 3 years old boy, my wife and I were careful with the food intake of our son. Discouraging him from eating sweet food at a young age will make him less prone to develop a sweet tooth when he grows up. Our children are also exposed to sugary food at school. We can't control much with his food intake at school, i.e. we can't tell him not to eat his friend's birthday cake at school. We just do our part to control his food intake at home.

If you must take sugar, you can use xylitol instead, which has the lowest Glycemic Index and won't trigger insulin spike

LOSING WEIGHT - WHY CALORIES LOSS COUNTS

Over recent years, the focus in weight loss programs has been largely low carb or low fat diets. In order to lose weight, you need to eat fewer calories than you need to use across each day. So regardless of what your diet or eating program is called, the bottom line about all successful weight loss is calories loss.

Are you ready to figure out how many calories you should take in each day? There are several ways to decide what your ideal calorie intake should be. Some are complicated and involve calculating your Base Metabolic Rate and then adding the amount of energy you normally put into physical activity, and adding in how efficiently your body processes food.

You can go to a nutritionist who has tools to measure those values and get a very precise figure of how many calories you should be eating each day. But if you want a simpler formula to figure out how many calories you should be taking in each day to keep your body functioning, there is an easier way. First, you need to assess your activity level.

You are sedentary if you sit at a computer all day and do no more physical activity than walking around the grocery store. The best way to figure out how many calories you need to take in on a daily basis is to take your weight and multiply it by 14, so if you weigh 150 pounds, you would multiply 150 x 14 and get 2100, so you need to take in 2,100 calories each day to maintain your weight. To lose weight through calories loss your intake will need to be less than this.

If you are moderately active, you don't work out every day but you might hit the gym two or three times a week or walk or bike ride around the neighborhood at night. To figure out how many calories you need each day, take your weight and multiply it by 17 so the total will give you the number of calories you should take in to maintain your weight. To lose weight through calories loss your intake will need to be less than this.

If you bike to work, go to the gym every day, or run five miles at night, you are active. In order to figure out your ideal calorie intake, multiply your weight by 20 and that is how many calories your body needs to keep working efficiently. To lose weight through calories loss your intake will need to be less than this.

A food diary is a great way to get an accurate idea of how many calories you consume in a day and figure out how many calories are in each of the things that you ate that day. There are lots of commercially available calorie counting books that give the total number of calories for a lot of common foods and even fast foods. Using a food diary you can accurately count the calories in a fast food meal and determine what and how much you can eat in order to lose weight through calories loss.

Counting calories may take a little time at the outset, but it becomes a lot easier and will help you control what you eat so you can lose weight and keep it off forever.

HOW TO COUNT CALORIES ACCORDING TO BODY WEIGHT

Your caloric intake is the most important factor in determining your weight. It comes down to how many calories you consume versus how many you burn. Both exercise and diet influence how effectively you burn calories. Whether your goal is to lose, gain or maintain weight, there is a method to calculate your daily calorie requirements. You will need to know your current level of physical activity, height and weight to use the equation.

1. Weigh yourself. Use a bathroom scale to determine your weight in pounds. A scale usually gives your weight in stones.

2. Calculate your basic metabolic rate (BMR). Your BMR is your resting metabolic rate, which is how active your metabolism is when you are not performing any physical activity, such as sleep. If you're a woman, use the following formula to calculate your BMR: 655 + (4.35 x weight in pounds) + (4.7 x height in inches) - (4.7 x age in years).

Use the following formula to calculate your BMR if you are a man: 66 + (6.23 x weight in pounds) + (12.7 x height in inches) - (6.8 x age in years). For example, a 23-year-old man who is 6 feet 2 inches tall, weighing 185 pounds, has a basic metabolic rate of 2,003.

3. Multiply your BMR by the level of physical activity you get. If you get little or no exercise, times your BMR by 1.2, and if you perform light exercise, such as walking one to three days a week, multiply your BMR by 1.375. For a moderate level of exercise, such as jogging three to five times a week, multiply your BMR by 1.55. And for those who are very active and exercise or engage in sports most days of the week, times your BMR by 1.725. Calculate an athletic level of exercise by multiplying your BMR by 1.9. The result is the ideal number of calories you should consume daily. The very active 23-year-old man in the example above would multiply his BMR by 1.725, for a total of 3,452 calories daily.

4. Increase your ideal number of calories by 500 to 1,000 daily to increase your weight by 1 to 2 pounds a week, or decrease your calories if you want to lose weight.

Things You Will Need

- Scale
- Calculator
- Tip

Read nutrition labels or use an online calorie counter to find out the amount of calories in each meal you consume. This will help you keep track of your caloric intake.

CHAPTER SIX: COMBINING INTERMITTENT FASTING AND KETOGENIC DIET

If you commit to the ketogenic diet while doing intermittent fasting as well, it could offer the following benefits.

-May Smooth Your Path to Ketosis

Intermittent fasting may help your body reach ketosis quicker than using the keto diet alone.

That's because your body, when fasting, maintains its energy balance by shifting its fuel source from carbs to fats — the exact premise of the keto diet.

During fasting, insulin levels and glycogen stores decrease, leading your body to naturally start burning fat for fuel.

For anyone who struggles to reach ketosis while on a keto diet, adding intermittent fasting may effectively jumpstart your process.

-May Lead to More Fat Loss

Combining the diet and the fast may help you burn more fat than the diet alone.

Because intermittent fasting boosts your metabolism by promoting thermogenesis, or heat production, your body may start utilizing stubborn fat stores.

Several studies have revealed that intermittent fasting can powerfully and safely drop excess body fat.

In an eight-week study in 34 resistance-trained men, those who practiced the 16/8 method of intermittent fasting lost nearly 14% more body fat than those following a normal eating pattern.

Similarly, a review of 28 studies noted that people who used intermittent fasting lost an average of 7.3 pounds (3.3 kg) more fat mass than those following very low-calorie diets.

Plus, intermittent fasting may preserve muscle mass during weight loss and improve energy levels, which may be helpful for keto dieters looking to improve athletic performance and drop body fat.

Additionally, studies underscore that intermittent fasting can reduce hunger and promote feelings of fullness, which may aid weight loss.

Combining the ketogenic diet with intermittent fasting is likely safe for most people.

However, pregnant or breastfeeding women and those with a history of disordered eating should avoid intermittent fasting.

People with certain health conditions, such as diabetes or heart disease, should consult with a doctor before trying intermittent fasting on the keto diet.

Though some people may find merging the practices helpful, it's important to note that it may not work for everyone.

Some people may find that fasting on the keto diet is too difficult, or they may experience adverse reactions, such as overeating on non-fasting days, irritability and fatigue.

Keep in mind that intermittent fasting is not necessary to reach ketosis, even though it can be used as a tool to do so quickly.

Simply following a healthy, well-rounded keto diet is enough for anyone looking to improve health by cutting down on carbs.

SMOOTHIES FOR KETO

You may be one of those people who has made the decision to lead a healthier lifestyle. Is that why you are looking for a bit of help? Are you here because you want to know more about how to make delicious and spectacular smoothies?

Smoothie information is so in-demand these days. But what makes smoothies special when they are just part purée and part fruit drink? They are easy to make, so much so that anyone can prepare one. It takes no special skill to concoct a foamy, fruity mix that you can enjoy by yourself or share with people close to you.

What makes smoothies a special type of beverage is that they can be so nutritious that you won't need to take multivitamins and other expensive supplements anymore if you include smoothies in your daily diet. Smoothies are very good for you.

There was a time when smoothies were novelties and specialities offered only in cafes, restaurants, and juice bars. Now you can make them at home. If you are new to the smoothie phenomenon, you can learn how to make a handful of basic preparations such as strawberry smoothies, banana smoothies, and mango smoothies. But you should realize that there is a whole new world of smoothie information that you have not yet glimpsed. Allow us to impart a few tips that you can use to make more refreshing, exciting, and very delicious smoothie preparations.

Smoothies are first and foremost an excellent way to get healthy. They allow you to meet your daily recommended servings of fruits and vegetables that many people lack in their diets. Smoothies allow you to create a drink using whole fruits and vegetables without discarding much of the fruit or vegetables as you would do if you ate the fruit or vegetable itself.

BENEFITS OF SMOOTHIES

Smoothies aren't only beverages that go with the new trend. They give benefits which are good to health at the same time.

Here are some benefits that smoothies contain:

1. Milk-Based Smoothies Provide Calcium - Smoothies that were made with dairy products give calcium for bone strength so that they will stay strong even into old age. Whole milk gives almost a third of your daily requirements of calcium. It also contains fats and vitamins to keep our body alive.

2. Smoothies Make A Healthy Breakfast More Convenient - A homemade smoothie for your morning meal is excellent. It gives you energy to maintain cheerfulness until the end of the day. Drinking a smoothie in the morning helps you stop indulging in empty carbohydrates. In fact, a nutritious smoothie does better when it comes to body enrichment that multivitamins do.

3. Good Smoothies Are Nutrient- Dense and Contain Fat - the best smoothies are nutrient - dense, providing vitamins and oils necessary for good nutrition. Fat is required for biological function and is burned by your body for energy; it also helps with the maintenance of our body.

4. Healthy Smoothies Are Simple To Make - Healthy smoothies are easy to produce. When you have a good blender and quality ingredients, you can now have a delicious, healthy smoothie in just a snap. It's not the thing that would consume a great amount of time but it helps you to create an instant but healthy beverage.

5. Smoothies Help You Keep Hydrated - A smoothie for breakfast helps you keep hydrated at the start of the day. A glass of smoothie will quench your thirst so you don't have to drink water every time you get thirsty.

Making and drinking these smoothies is a good habit for every day and is a great replacement for sodas and any other forms of beverages which don't have positive nutritional effects on the body.

BASIC COMPONENTS OF A SMOOTHIE

If you're going to try your hand at making your own smoothies, there are a few things you need to know. Smoothie ingredients break down into three categories: fruit, liquid and additions. Let's look at each of these in turn.

First, let's talk about fruit. Fruit forms the foundation of your smoothie. The fruit flavor will usually dominate, so you can pick your favorite fruits to give your smoothie its primary flavour identity. Now, not all fruit actually works in smoothies. Some fruits do well, others do horribly.

Creamy fruits, berries and stone fruits like peaches all work well in smoothies. Melons can work well in small amounts (or you can blend up a bunch of melon with other ingredients for one of your wilder smoothie experiments). However, lots of popular fruits don't work particularly well in smoothies. Apples, for instance, don't really make great smoothie foundation material. Use apple cider as a liquid base instead for an apple-flavoured smoothie.

Since there are so many different types of fruits, I can't really tell you which ones will work and which ones won't on a case by case basis. Just be aware that some of the fruits you add to your smoothies might not actually end up working well. And that's totally okay.

Once you've chosen your fruit, you need to add in a liquid. Juices work really well. Water tends to be a little tricky because your smoothie can easily end up quite tasteless. It's weird how you can have tons of fruits and other ingredients, but water's dilutional power simply takes the edge off of all the flavors. My personal favorite (current) smoothie liquid is coconut water.

You can find it at some health food stores, or do what I do and order it directly from Amazon for a discount.

Finally, no smoothie would be complete without some extra ingredients. This is where the sky really is the limit. You can add nutritional supplements (particularly the powdered kind), nuts (use raw nuts or be prepared to ruin your nut addition) and leafy greens (spinach, kale and parsley are fantastic but use these with care lest your smoothie be more nutritious than actually tasty).

HOW TO MAKE SMOOTHIES

Using The Right Equipment To Make The Perfect Smoothie

Most people prefer learning how to make smoothies with a good quality smoothie blender. While there are cheaper ones available in the market, they have limited functions. A marvelous blender will allow you to make the best smoothies with just the right texture.

Ingredients To Liquefy Your Smoothie

There are a few basic building blocks when it comes time to make a smoothie. The first essential ingredient is the liquid or thinning agent. Liquids like fresh milk, cow's milk, and soy milk are great options. These will offer you a dose of calcium, protein, and contains flavones. While fruit juices can also be used, they generally have a high sugar content and if your intention is to learn how to make smoothies that are nutritional, you would do better to skip the fruit juice and stick to soy milk instead.

Fresh Produce

To this liquid, you must add your choice of fruits and vegetables. These change the taste as well as the texture of your smoothie. Pick tastes that blend well together. You can keep mixing and matching to find the smoothie that you like best. In your journey of how to make smoothies that are delicious as well as healthy, feel free to use fruits like strawberries, blackberries, apples, kiwis, cherries, grapes, and vegetables like pumpkin, and raw spinach! These ingredients pack a powerful punch and are full of nutritional value.

Thickening Ingredient

The next step in learning how to make smoothies is to add a thickener to the mixture. This can be added in the form of ice crushed, cubes, and frozen fruit depending on the strength and capacity of your blender. Frozen fruits can also be used as a thickening agent but again you will need a powerful blender that will purify them. This ingredient adds to the texture and consistency of the smoothie.

While learning how to make smoothies, you need to realize that this is a process that is flexible and depends entirely on your taste and preferences. If you prefer your smoothies a little runny, consider using less of the thickener and more of the milk or juice. If the smoothies turn out to be too thin, simply add more frozen fruits or ice. If you feel like your smoothie is too watered down, add some more fruit to it. If you want to add a little more flavor to it, add some cinnamon or honey.

To achieve the right consistency, most blenders take within 30 to 45 seconds to fully chop up or blend the ingredients. Allow your smoothie to circulate freely without any lumps inside the blender for at least 5 to 10 seconds before you consider it ready. Now you've learned how to make smoothies!

Since each of those three categories contains a near-infinite potential for variation, you can see that the number of total smoothies is basically infinite. Don't be afraid to mix up something strange! Instead, be brave, get out your blender and have at it--it's smoothie time!

SMOOTHIE RECIPES FOR WEIGHT LOSS

Many people wonder if the smoothie diet will work to help them lose weight. If you follow the right plan, the weight can come off pretty darn quick for you too.

The smoothie method for losing weight is essentially a low-calorie diet where you substitute your usual meals with fruit or vegetable smoothies.

For smoothie enthusiasts - let me tell you - when you do this, it will not feel like you are dieting at all. You will not feel deprived as you do on most diets.

And if you do it right you won't suffer from those awful hunger pains. This is not a starvation diet - this is a healthy, nutritious, delicious meal replacement diet that you do short term to supercharge weight loss and flood your body with living foods that give you lots of nutrition and vitamins.

So how does drinking smoothies help you lose weight? Smoothies, when made correctly and nutritiously, can fill you up so you are NOT hungry and you won't be tempted to eat forbidden high-calorie foods.

Can you lose weight fast? It depends.... if you follow the wrong plan you may end up drinking smoothies that are high calorie and low in nutritional value. You know, it is the same way that you can ruin a healthy salad by pouring half a container of high-fat dressing on it. With this in mind, I've put together these simple, healthy recipes for weight loss that will have you on your way to dropping those pounds quickly.

These recipes will not only allow you to feel full during fasting, but are also suitable for weightloss.

1. Low Carb Acai Almond Butter Smoothie

Servings: 1

Ingredients:

- 1 100g pack unsweetened acai puree
- 3/4 cup unsweetened almond milk
- 1/4 of an avocado
- 3 tbsp collagen or protein powder
- 1 tbsp coconut oil or MCT oil powder
- 1 tbsp almond butter
- 1/2 tsp vanilla extract
- 2 drops liquid stevia (optional)

Instructions:

- If you are using individualized 100 gram packs of acai puree, run the pack under lukewarm water for a few seconds until you are able to break up the puree into smaller pieces. Open the pack and put the contents into the blender.
- Place the remaining ingredients in the blender and blend until smooth. Add more water or ice cubes as needed.

- Drizzle the almond butter along the side of the glass to make it look cool.
- Enjoy and pat yourself on the back for an awesome workout and killer post workout smoothie!

Nutritional Values:

- Calories: 345 Kcal
- Fat: 20g
- Carbohydrates: 8g
- Fiber: 2g
- Protein: 15g

2. Keto Blueberry Smoothie

Servings: 1

This keto smoothie is perfect for a quick breakfast or a post-workout refuel option. It's packed with antioxidants for better detoxification, Vitamin C for a healthy immune system, and folate for proper cholesterol function.

Ingredients:

- 1 cup coconut milk or almond milk
- 1/4 cup blueberries
- 1 tsp vanilla extract
- 1 tsp MCT oil or coconut oil
- 30 g protein powder (optional)

Instructions:

- Put all the ingredients into a blender, and blend until smooth.

Notes

If you like the swirl, you can add a tablespoon of full-fat yogurt after the smoothie is in the cup and swirl it around, touching the sides.

Suitable Substitutions

MCT Oil - If you don't have any MCT oil that's totally fine, you can replace this with coconut oil or any fat you like.

Blueberries - Any berry will work (blackberry, raspberry, strawberry) and will have a similar carbohydrate content.

Protein Powder - If you don't have protein powder, you can simply omit this from the recipe. If you still want a fluffy texture you could try adding a raw egg, but these can sometimes contain salmonella so pregnant women should avoid this.

Milk Alternatives - you can make this with unsweetened almond milk, unsweetened coconut milk, pea milk, and they all taste similar; just find milk you like, and use that.

Nutritional Values:

- Calories: 215 Kcal
- Fat: 10g
- Carbohydrates: 7g
- Fiber: 3g
- Protein: 23g

3. Minty Green Protein Smoothie (Dairy Free & Low Carb)

Servings: 1

Ingredients:

- 1/2 of an avocado
- 1 cup fresh spinach
- 10-12 drops SweetLeaf® Liquid Stevia Peppermint Sweet Drops™
- 1 scoop Whey Protein Powder
- 1/2 cup unsweetened almond milk
- 1/4 tsp peppermint extract
- 1 cup ice
- Optional: cacao nibs

Instructions:

- Place avocado, spinach, protein powder and milk in a blender and blend until smooth. Add the SweetLeaf® Liquid Stevia Peppermint Sweet Drops™, extract, and ice, and blend until thick. Taste and adjust stevia, as needed.

Nutritional Values:

- Net carbs: 4g
- Calories: 293 Kcal
- Fat: 15g
- Fiber: 7g
- Protein: 28

4. Turmeric Keto Smoothie

Servings: 1

Ingredients:

- 200 ml full fat coconut milk
- 200 ml unsweetened almond milk
- 1 tsp granulated sweetener (stevia etc.) or other sweetener
- 1 tbsp ground turmeric
- 1 tsp ground cinnamon
- 1 tsp ground ginger
- 1 tbsp MCT oil or use coconut oil
- 1 tbsp chia seeds to top

Instructions:

- Combine all the ingredients except the chia seeds in a blender, add some ice and blend until smooth.
- Sprinkle chia seeds on top and enjoy!

Nutritional Values:

- Fat: 56g
- Protein: 7g
- Net Carbs: 6g
- Calories: 600 Kcal

5. Raspberry Avocado Smoothie - Dairy Free

Servings: 2

Ingredients:

- 1 ripe avocado, peeled and with pit removed
- 1 1/3 cup water
- 2-3 tablespoons lemon juice
- 2 tbsp low carb sugar substitute - I like to use 1/8 teaspoon liquid stevia extract
- 1/2 cup frozen unsweetened raspberries or other low carb frozen berries

Instructions:

- Add all ingredients to blender.

- Blend until smooth.
- Pour into two tall glasses and enjoy with a straw!

Nutritional Values per serving:

- Net carbs: 4g
- Calories: 227 kcal
- Fat: 20g
- Fiber: 8.8g
- Protein: 2.5g

6. Mean Green Matcha Protein Shake

Matcha powder, protein powder, almond milk, and leafy greens make up this matcha protein shake. Have it as a breakfast smoothie or a pre-workout snack for the energy boost you crave.

Servings: 1

Ingredients:

- 1 cup unsweetened milk of choice
- ¼ cup coconut milk
- 1 scoop Perfect Keto Unflavored Whey Protein Powder or vanilla protein powder
- 1 scoop Perfect Keto Matcha MCT oil powder
- 1 large handful spinach
- 1 small avocado

- 1 tablespoon coconut oil
- 1 cup of ice (optional)

Instructions:

- Add all ingredients to a high-speed blender and mix on high until smooth.
- Garnish with chopped mint leaves and a few berries if desired.

Nutritional Values:

- Calories: 334 Kcal
- Fat: 24g
- Carbohydrates: 13g
- Fiber: 10g
- Protein: 19g

7. Keto Beetroot Shake

Servings: 1

Ingredients:

- 1 tsp Temple Nutrition Beetroot Powder
- 1 tbsp Temple Nutrition MCT Oil (use 1 tsp if you are new to MCT oil)
- 1 scoop Whey Protein Isolate (Optional)
- 1 tsp vanilla extract

- 1/4 tsp cinnanmon, ground
- 1 cup coconut milk or almond milk, pea milk

Instructions:

- Put all ingredients into a high speed blender.
- Blend for 30 seconds.
- Pour into a glass, or drink straight from the container. Top with extra beetroot powder if desired.

Nutritional Values:

- Calories: 300 Kcal
- Fat: 19g
- Carbohydrates: 6g
- Fiber: 3g
- Protein 25g

KETO RECIPES

KETO BREAKFAST RECIPES

1. Keto Coffee Recipe – 4 Variations

Prep Time: 2 Minutes
Cook Time: 5 Minutes
Total Time: 7 Minutes

Servings: 1

Keto Coffee Recipe – Variation 1 – Traditional

Ingredients:

- 1 cup (240 ml) black coffee
- 1/2 teaspoon (2 ml) MCT oil (add more once you know you can handle it!)
- 1 Tablespoon (15 ml) ghee

Nutritional Values per serving:

- Calories: 143 Kcal
- Fat: 17g
- Net Carbs: 0g
- Protein: 0g

Keto Coffee Recipe – Variation 2 – Coconut

Ingredients:

- 1 cup (240 ml) of black coffee
- 1/2 Tablespoon (7 ml) coconut oil
- 1 Tablespoon (15 ml) ghee

Nutritional Values per serving:

- Calories: 179 Kcal
- Fat: 21g

- Net Carbs: 0g
- Protein: 0g

Keto Coffee Recipe – Variation 3 – Frothy

Ingredients:

- 1 cup (240 ml) of black coffee
- 1/2 Tablespoon (7 ml) coconut oil
- 1 Tablespoon (15 ml) ghee
- 2 Tablespoons (30 ml) unsweetened coconut or almond milk

Nutritional Values per serving:

- Calories: 190 Kcal
- Fat: 22g
- Net Carbs: 0g
- Protein: 0g

Keto Coffee Recipe – Variation 4 – Collagen Boosted

Ingredients:

- 1 cup (240 ml) of black coffee
- 1 Tablespoon (15 ml) ghee
- 1/2 scoop unflavored hydrolyzed collagen powder (try CoBionic Indulgence to add a mocha flavor to your coffee!)

Nutritional Values per serving:

- Calories: 160 Kcal
- Fat: 14g
- Net Carbs: 0g
- Protein: 5g

Instructions:

- Combine all ingredients in a blender. Pour into a coffee mug to serve.

2. Keto Chocolate Hazelnut Muffins Recipe (Dairy-Free)

Prep Time: 10 Minutes

Cook Time: 20 Minutes

Total Time: 30 Minutes

Yield: 12 Muffins

Ingredients:

- 3 cups (360 g) almond flour
- 1/2 cup (120 ml) coconut oil, melted
- 4 large eggs, whisked
- 1/2 teaspoon nutmeg
- 1/4 teaspoon cloves
- 1/2 cup (100 g) hazelnuts, chopped
- Low carb sweetener of choice (we recommend Stevia), to taste

- Dash of salt
- 1 teaspoon (8 g) baking soda
- 3 oz (80 g) 100% dark chocolate, broken into chunks

Instructions:

- Preheat oven to 350 F (175 C).
- Mix together the almond flour, coconut oil, eggs, nutmeg, cloves, chopped hazelnuts, sweetener, salt, and baking soda.
- Pour the mixture into 12 lined or greased muffin pans.
- Place chocolate chunks on the top each muffin, pressing them down into the dough/mixture.
- Bake for 18-20 minutes so that a toothpick comes out clean when you insert it into a muffin.

Nutritional Values per serving:

Serving Size: 1 muffin

- Calories: 282 Kcal
- Sugar: 1g
- Fat: 25g
- Carbohydrates: 6g
- Fiber: 3g
- Protein: 8g

3. Easy Breakfast Baked Egg in Avocado

Prep Time: 5 Minutes

Cook Time: 12 Minutes

Total Time: 17 Minutes

Servings: 2

Ingredients:

- 1 avocado
- 2 egg yolks
- 2 teaspoons olive oil or coconut oil
- Salt and pepper and other seasoning/spices/herbs to taste (smoked paprika goes well with eggs)

Instructions:

- Preheat oven to 400 F (200 C).
- Slice the avocado in half and remove the stone.
- Crack the 2 eggs into a bowl.
- Scoop out each egg yolk and place each into an avocado half.
- Pour 1 teaspoon of olive oil onto each egg yolk in the avocado.
- Bake for 12 minutes.
- Sprinkle salt and pepper and whatever additional herbs and spices you'd like on top.

Nutritional Values per serving:

- Calories: 250 Kcal
- Sugar: 1g
- Fat: 23g
- Carbohydrates: 9g
- Fiber: 7g
- Protein: 3g

4. Keto Breakfast Stack

Prep Time: 15 Minutes
Cook Time: 15 Minutes
Total Time: 30 Minutes
Servings: 2

Ingredients:

- 4 slices bacon (use AIP-compliant bacon if you're staying AIP)
- 1/4 lb (110 g) ground pork
- 1/4 lb (110 g) ground chicken
- 2 teaspoons (2 g) Italian seasoning
- 1 egg, whisked (omit for AIP)
- 1 teaspoon (5 g) salt
- 1/4 teaspoon black pepper (omit for AIP)
- 2 large flat mushrooms (like portobello)
- 1 avocado, sliced

Instructions:

- Cook the bacon until crispy. Leave the fat in the pan.
- Mix together the ground pork, chicken, Italian seasoning, egg, salt, and pepper in a bowl and form 4 thin patties.
- Pan-fry the patties in the bacon fat.
- Then pan-fry the mushrooms.
- Put together your keto breakfast stack with the mushrooms on the bottom, then 2 thin patties, then 3 slices of avocado, and top it with the slices of bacon. Serve with the rest of the avocado slices.

Nutritional Values per serving:

- Calories: 680 Kcal
- Sugar: 2g
- Fat: 54g
- Carbohydrates: 13g
- Fiber: 8g
- Protein: 38g

5. Paleo Chicken and Bacon Sausages

Prep Time: 10 Minutes
Cook Time: 20 Minutes
Total Time: 30 Minutes
Servings: 12

Ingredients:

- 2 large chicken breasts, or use 1 lb ground chicken
- 2 slices bacon, cooked and broken into small bits
- 1 egg, whisked (omit for AIP)
- 2 tablespoons Italian seasoning
- 2 teaspoons garlic powder
- 2 teaspoons onion powder
- Salt and pepper

Instructions:

- In a large skillet, melt the coconut oil over a medium-high heat. Add the turkey and bacon to the skillet and sauté until slightly browned – for about 5 to 7 minutes.
- Add the onion, asparagus, spinach and fresh thyme to the skillet. Sauté for an additional 10 minutes until the turkey and bacon are cooked through and the vegetables are soft.
- Season with salt and pepper, to taste.

Nutritional Values per serving:

- Calories: 370 Kcal
- Sugar: 1g
- Fat: 21g
- Carbohydrates: 3g
- Fiber: 1g
- Protein: 40g

6. Almond Flour Pancakes (Keto-friendly)

Prep Time: 5 Minutes

Cook Time: 15 Minutes

Total Time: 20 Minutes

Servings: 6

Ingredients:

- 1 cup blanched almond flour
- 2 eggs
- 2 tablespoons maple syrup (optional; or use water)
- 2 tablespoons olive oil (or any other liquid oil)
- 1 teaspoon baking powder
- 1 teaspoon vanilla extract
- 1/4 teaspoon fine sea salt

Instructions:

Skillet Pancakes:

- Preheat a skillet over a medium-low heat on the stove. As it heats, stir together the almond flour, eggs, maple syrup (if using), olive oil, baking powder, vanilla, and salt in a large bowl. The batter will be a little thicker than traditional pancake batter.
- Grease the preheated skillet with butter or olive oil, then pour 3 to 4 tablespoons of the batter into the

center of the skillet (I use a scant 1/4 cup). Use a spatula to spread the batter out into a round pancake shape, about 1/4 to 1/2-inch thick.

- Cook until little bubbles start to form around the edges of the pancake, and as soon as the bottom feels sturdy enough to flip (about 3 to 4 minutes of cooking time), use a spatula to flip the pancake and cook the other side, about 2 to 3 more minutes.

- Repeat with the remaining batter, until all of the pancakes are cooked. I usually get about 6 pancakes from this batch that are roughly 4 to 6 inches in diameter. Even though they are on the smaller side, they are very filling! Serve warm with your favorite toppings.

Oven-Baked Pancakes:

- Prepare the batter as directed above, but instead of using the stove, preheat the oven to 350ºF and line a large baking sheet with parchment paper.

- Pour the prepared batter by a scant 1/4 cup onto the lined baking sheet, and use a spoon or spatula to spread the batter into a round pancake shape until it's 1/4-inch thick. Leave about 1 inch between each pancake, and repeat with the remaining batter until you have roughly 6 pancakes on the pan.

- Bake at 350ºF for 10 minutes. The pancakes should puff up, and you don't need to flip them as long as they look like they are thoroughly cooked through. I like to flip them over for serving, so the browned side is on top. Serve warm, with your favorite pancake toppings.

Nutrional values per serving:

Made with maple syrup:

- Calories: 193 Kcal
- Fat: 15g
- Carbohydrates: 9g
- Fiber: 1.5g
- Protein: 6g

Made without syrup:

- Calories: 175 Kcal
- Fat: 15g
- Carbohydrates: 4g
- Fiber: 1g
- Protein: 6g

KETO LUNCH AND DINNER RECIPES

1. Bacon and Avocado Caesar Salad

Prep Time: 10 Minutes
Cook Time: 5 Minutes

Total Time: 15 Minutes

Servings: 2

Ingredients:

For the salad:

- 4 slices of bacon (112 g), diced
- 1 head of romaine lettuce (200 g), chopped
- 1/2 cucumber (110 g), thinly sliced
- 1/4 medium onion (28 g), thinly sliced
- 1 large avocado (200 g), sliced

For the Caesar dressing:

- 1/4 cup of mayo (60 ml)
- 1 tablespoon of lemon juice (15 ml)
- 1 teaspoon of Dijon mustard (5 ml)
- 1 teaspoon of garlic powder (3.5 g)
- Salt and pepper, to taste

Instructions:

- Add the bacon to a large nonstick skillet over medium-high heat and sauté until crispy, for about 5 minutes. Remove the bacon from the skillet with a slotted spoon and place on a paper towel lined plate to cool.

- In a small bowl, whisk to combine the mayo, lemon juice, mustard, and garlic powder. Season with salt and pepper, to taste.
- Toss the remaining Caesar dressing with the romaine lettuce leaves. Add the cucumber and onion to the bowl and toss to combine.
- Divide the salad between 2 plates and top each salad with equal amounts of cooked bacon and sliced avocado.

Nutritional Values per serving:

- Calories: 652 Kcal
- Sugar: 3g
- Fat: 65g
- Carbohydrates: 15g
- Fiber: 9g
- Protein: 10g

2. Lemon Garlic Ghee Keto Salmon Recipe with Leek Asparagus Ginger Saute

Prep Time: 10 Minutes

Cook Time: 20 Minutes

Total Time: 30 Minutes

Servings: 2

Ingredients:

For the lemon garlic ghee salmon:

- 2 fillets of salmon (with skin on), fresh or frozen (340 g), defrost if frozen
- 1 tablespoon (15 ml) ghee (use avocado oil for AIP)
- 4 cloves garlic (12 g), minced
- 2 teaspoons (10 ml) lemon juice
- Salt to taste
- Lemon slices to serve with

For the leek asparagus ginger sauté:

- 10 spears of asparagus (160 g), chopped into small pieces
- 1 leek (90 g), chopped into small pieces
- 2 teaspoons (4 g) ginger powder (or use finely diced fresh ginger if you have it available)
- Avocado oil or olive oil to sauté with
- 1 Tablespoon lemon juice
- Salt to taste

Instructions:

- Preheat oven to 400 F (200 C).
- Place each salmon fillet on a piece of aluminum foil or parchment paper.
- Divide the ghee, lemon juice and minced garlic between the two fillets – place these on top of the salmon.

Sprinkle with some salt. Then wrap up the salmon in the foil and place into the oven.

- Open up the foil after 10 minutes in the oven and then bake for another 10 minutes.
- While the salmon is cooking, place 1-2 tablespoons of avocado oil or olive oil into a frying pan and sauté the chopped asparagus and leek on a high heat. Saute for 10 minutes and then add in the ginger powder, lemon juice, and salt to taste. Saute for 1 more minute.
- Serve by dividing the sauté between 2 plates and placing a salmon fillet on top of each.

Nutritional Values per serving:

- Calories: 680 Kcal
- Sugar: 4g
- Fat: 51g
- Carbohydrates: 15g
- Fiber: 4g
- Protein: 30g

3. Lemon Black Pepper Tuna Salad Recipe

Prep Time: 10 Minutes

Cook Time: 0 Minutes

Total Time: 10 Minutes

Servings: 1

Ingredients:

- 1/3 cucumber, diced small
- 1/2 small avocado, diced small
- 1 teaspoon lemon juice
- 1 can (4-6 oz or 100–150 g) of tuna
- 1 tablespoon Paleo mayo (use olive oil for AIP)
- 1 tablespoon mustard (omit for AIP)
- Salt to taste
- Salad greens (optional)
- Black pepper to taste (omit for AIP)

Instructions:

- Mix together the diced cucumber and avocado with the lemon juice.
- Flake the tuna and mix well with the mayo and mustard.
- Add the tuna to the avocado and cucumber. Add salt to taste.
- Prepare the salad greens (optional: add olive oil and lemon juice to taste).
- Place the tuna salad on top of the salad greens.
- Sprinkle black pepper on top.

Nutritional Values per serving:

- Calories: 480 Kcal
- Sugar: 2g

- Fat: 40g
- Carbohydrates: 11g
- Fiber: 8g
- Protein: 45g

4. Paleo Pressure Cooker Beef And Broccoli

Prep Time: 5 Minutes

Cook Time: 15 Minutes

Total Time: 20 Minutes

Servings: 2

Ingredients:

- 1 tablespoon (15 ml) of olive oil
- 14 oz (400 g) of beef sirloin, cut into bite-size pieces
- 1 teaspoon (2 g) of ginger paste (or minced fresh ginger)
- 1 teaspoon (2 g) of garlic paste (or 1 minced garlic clove)
- 1/2 cup (120 ml) of beef broth
- 1 1/2 tablespoons (23 ml) of gluten-free tamari sauce (or coconut aminos)
- 1/2 head (8 oz or 225 g) of broccoli, broken into small florets
- 1 teaspoon (5 ml) of honey
- Salt and pepper, to taste

Instructions:

- Add the olive oil and beef to the pressure cooker and sauté until browned. Add the ginger paste and garlic paste and sauté for a few seconds. Add the beef broth, tamari sauce, and broccoli to the pressure cooker, stirring to combine.
- Secure the lid on the pressure cooker to close. Set the pressure cooker to cook for 10 minutes and then let the pressure release naturally before removing the lid carefully.
- Remove the beef and broccoli from the pressure cooker with a slotted spoon and set aside to keep warm. To create a sauce, add the honey to the pressure cooker and reduce the liquid by half. Season with salt and pepper, to taste.
- To serve, place the beef and broccoli on 2 plates and spoon equal amounts of the sauce over each plate.

Nutritional Values per serving:

- Calories: 643 Kcal
- Sugar: 4g
- Fat: 49g
- Carbohydrates: 10g
- Fiber: 4g
- Protein: 37g

5. Keto Cottage Pie

Prep Time: 15 Minutes

Cook Time: 1 Hour

Total Time: 1 Hour, 15 Minutes

Servings: 10

Ingredients:

Base:

- 3 tablespoons olive oil
- 2 cloves garlic crushed
- 1 tablespoon dried oregano
- 1 small onion diced
- 3 sticks celery diced
- 1 teaspoon salt
- 2 pounds ground beef
- 3 tablespoons tomato paste
- 1 cup beef stock
- 1/4 cup red wine vinegar
- 2 tablespoons fresh thyme leaves
- 10 ounces green beans, cut into 1in lengths

Topping:

- 1.6 pounds cauliflower cut into florets
- 3 ounces butter

- 1/2 teaspoon salt
- 1/4 teaspoon pepper
- 3 egg yolks
- Pinch paprika
- Pinch dried oregano

Instructions:

Base:

- Place a large saucepan over a high heat.
- Add the olive oil, garlic, oregano, onion and celery and Sauté for 5 minutes, until the onion is starting to become translucent.
- Add the salt and ground beef, stirring continuously to break apart the meat while it browns.
- When the beef is browned add the tomato paste and stir well.
- Add the beef stock and red wine vinegar and simmer uncovered for 20 minutes until the liquid has reduced.
- Add the thyme and green beans and simmer for 5 minutes before removing from the heat.
- Spoon the beef mixture into your casserole dish and set aside.
- Preheat your oven to 175C/350F.

Topping:

- Fill a large saucepan two-thirds full of water and bring to the boil.
- Add the cauliflower and cook for 7-10 minutes until tender.
- Carefully pour the water and cauliflower into a colander and drain well.
- Return the drained cauliflower to the saucepan, along with the butter, salt and pepper.
- Using your stick blender, blend the cauliflower into a smooth mash.
- Add the egg yolks and blend well.
- Gently spoon the mashed cauliflower onto the beef mixture in your casserole dish.
- Sprinkle with paprika and oregano.
- Bake the pie in the oven for 25-30 minutes, until the mash is golden brown.
- Serve immediately or chill and store in the fridge for up to 1 week.

Nutritional Values per serving:

Serving Size: 210g

- Calories: 420 Kcal
- Carbohydrates: 8g
- Protein: 18g
- Fat: 36g

- Fiber: 4g

6. Paleo Spanish Omelette

Prep Time: 15 minutes

Cook Time: 30 minutes

Totale Time: 45 Minutes

Servings: 4

Ingredients:

- 3 tablespoons of olive oil (45 ml), to cook with
- 2 medium bell peppers (240 g), diced
- 1 medium onion (110 g), diced
- 1/2 head of cauliflower (300 g), chopped
- 8 medium eggs, whisked
- 1/4 cup (60 ml) coconut cream
- 4 tablespoons (4 g) parsley, chopped
- Salt and pepper, to taste

Instructions:

- Preheat oven to 350 F (175 C).
- Sauté the bell pepper and onion with the olive oil. Season with salt and pepper to taste. Parboil the cauliflower florets – boil for 2 minutes and drain immediately.

- Mix the eggs, bell pepper, onion, cauliflower, coconut cream, and parsley together in a mixing bowl.
- Pour the mixture into a greased 9-inch by 9-inch (23-cm by 23-cm) square baking dish.
- Make sure to spread the vegetables (especially the cauliflower) out carefully.
- Bake for 20 minutes until the eggs are soft but set.

Nutritional Values per serving:

- Calories: 286 Kcal
- Sugar: 5g
- Fat: 22g
- Carbohydrates: 10g
- Fiber: 3g
- Protein: 14g

7. Simple Paleo Egg Salad

Prep Time: 5 Minutes
Cook Time: 15 Minutes
Total Time: 20 Minutes
Servings: 2

Ingredients:

- 4 hard boiled eggs, peeled
- 1/2 tablespoon mustard (add more to taste)

- 1/2 tablespoon mayo (optional – see here for a recipe or here to buy this Paleo mayo online)
- [Optional] 1 tablespoon pickles, chopped
- Salt to taste

Instructions:

- Cut up the hard boiled eggs into small pieces.
- In a bowl, combine with the mustard, mayo, and salt. Mix well.

Nutritional Values per serving:

- Calories: 268 Kcal
- Fat: 16g
- Carbohydrates: 6g
- Fiber: 1g
- Protein: 22g

8. Pan-Fried Tuscan Chicken Pasta

Prep Time: 10 Minutes

Cook Time: 10 Minutes

Total Time: 20 Minutes

Servings: 2

Ingredients:

- 2 chicken breasts, diced

- 2 small egg, whisked
- 1/4 teaspoon salt
- Dash of black pepper
- 2 teaspoons garlic powder
- 2 teaspoons Italian seasoning
- 14 cherry tomatoes, cut into quarters
- 30 basil leaves
- Olive oil or avocado oil to cook in
- Additional salt and pepper to taste
- 1 zucchini, peeled and turned into shreds or strands for the pasta

Instructions:

- In a bowl, mix together the whisked egg, salt, pepper, garlic powder, and Italian seasoning.
- Place the diced chicken pieces into the egg mixture and make sure the chicken is well covered with the mixture.
- Place 2 tablespoons of olive or avocado oil into a frying pan and sauté the chicken pieces coated with the egg mixture until the chicken pieces are fully cooked.
- Add in the quartered cherry tomatoes and fresh basil leaves. Sauté for 2-3 minutes more.
- Make the zucchini noodles by peeling a zucchini and then using the shredding attachment of a food processor or else using a potato peeler to create pasta-like strands or shreds.

- Divide the zucchini noodles into two and place onto plates. Top with the sautéed chicken.

Nutritional Values per serving:

- Calories: 540 Kcal
- Sugar: 4g
- Fat: 36g
- Carbohydrates: 7g
- Fiber: 2g
- Protein: 45g

9. Garlic Shrimp Caesar Salad

Prep Time: 15 Minutes
Cook Time: 10 Minutes
Total Time: 25 Minutes
Servings: 4

Ingredients:

For the shrimp:

- 1 lb shrimp (shells removed)
- 2 tablespoons olive oil
- 1 tablespoon lemon juice
- 3 tablespoons garlic powder
- 1 tablespoon onion powder

- Salt and pepper

For the salad:

- 1 head romaine lettuce, chopped
- 1 cucumber, chopped into cubes

For the dressing:

- 1 teaspoon Dijon mustard
- 1/4 cup Paleo mayo (you can purchase this one or make this one)
- 1 tablespoon fresh lemon juice
- 2 teaspoons garlic powder
- Salt and pepper

For garnish:

- 1 tablespoon parsley, chopped – for garnish
- 1 tablespoon sliced almonds – for garnish

Instructions:

- Preheat oven to 400F.
- Mix the shrimp, olive oil, lemon juice, garlic, onion powder, salt and pepper together. Place shrimp on baking tray and roast for 10 minutes.
- To make the salad dressing, blend the mayo, mustard, lemon juice, garlic powder, salt and pepper together.

- Toss the dressing with the chopped lettuce, chopped cucumber, and roasted shrimp. Garnish with the chopped parsley and sliced almonds.

Nutritional Values per serving:

Serving Size: 330 g

- Calories: 296 Kcal
- Sugar: 2g
- Fat: 19g
- Carbohydrates: 7g
- Fiber: 4g
- Protein: 25g

10. Zucchini noodles with avocado sauce

Prep time: 10 mins
Total time: 10 mins
Servings: 2

These delicious zucchini noodles (or zoodles) with avocado sauce are ready in 10 minutes. Besides, this recipe requires just 7 ingredients to make.

Ingredients:

- 1 zucchini
- 1 1/4 cup basil (30 g)

- 1/3 cup water (85 ml)
- 4 tbsp pine nuts
- 2 tbsp lemon juice
- 1 avocado
- 12 sliced cherry tomatoes

Instructions:

- Make the zucchini noodles using a peeler or the Spiralizer.
- Blend the rest of the ingredients (except the cherry tomatoes) in a blender until smooth.
- Combine noodles, avocado sauce and cherry tomatoes in a mixing bowl.
- These zucchini noodles with avocado sauce are better fresh, but you can store them in the fridge for 1 to 2 days.

Recipe Notes:

Feel free to use any veggies or fresh herbs you have on hand. You can also spiralize other veggies like carrots, beet, butternut squash, cabbage, etc.

Any nuts can be used instead of the pine nuts, or even seeds.

Nutritional Values per serving:

- Calories: 313 Kcal

- Sugar: 6.5g
- Fat: 26.8g
- Carbohydrates: 18.7g
- Fiber: 9.7g
- Protein: 6.8g

11. Paleo Chicken Noodle Soup Recipe

Prep Time: 15 Minutes

Cook Time: 15 Minutes

Total Time: 30 Minutes

Yield: 2 bowls

Ingredients:

- 3 cups chicken broth (use this recipe or buy this one) (approx 720ml)
- 1 chicken breast, chopped into small pieces (approx 240g or 0.5 lb)
- 2 tablespoons avocado oil
- 1 stalk of celery, chopped (approx 57g)
- 1 green onion, chopped (approx 10g)
- 1/4 cup cilantro, finely chopped (approx 15g)
- 1 zucchini, peeled (approx 106g)
- Salt to taste

Instructions:

- Dice the chicken breast.
- Add the avocado oil into a saucepan and sauté the diced chicken in there until cooked.
- Add chicken broth to the same saucepan and simmer.
- Chop the celery and add it into the saucepan.
- Chop the green onions and add them into the saucepan.
- Chop the cilantro and put it aside for the moment.
- Create zucchini noodles – I used a potato peeler to create long strands, but other options include using a spiralizer or a food processor with the shredding attachment.
- Add zucchini noodles and cilantro to the pot.
- Simmer for a few more minutes, add salt to taste, and serve immediately.

Nutritional Values per serving (1 bowl):

- Calories: 310 Kcal
- Sugar: 3g
- Fat: 16g
- Carbohydrates: 6g
- Fiber: 2g
- Protein: 34g

12. Keto Beef Teriyaki Recipe with Sesame and Kale

Prep Time: 10 Minutes

Cook Time: 10 Minutes

Total Time: 20 Minutes

Servings: 2

Ingredients:

- 2 tablespoons of gluten-free tamari sauce or coconut aminos (30 ml)
- 1 tablespoon of applesauce (15 ml)
- 2 cloves of garlic (6 g), minced
- 1 tablespoon of fresh ginger (4 g), minced
- 2 beef sirloin steaks (400 g) (pick a well marbled steak), sliced
- 1 tablespoon of sesame seeds (14 g)
- 1 teaspoon of sesame oil (5 ml)
- 2 tablespoons of avocado oil (30 ml)
- 10 white button mushrooms (100 g), sliced
- 2 oz of curly kale (56 g)
- Salt and pepper, to taste

Instructions:

- Whisk the tamari sauce, applesauce, garlic and ginger together in a bowl. Add the sliced sirloin and leave to marinate while you prep the remaining ingredients.
- Toast the sesame seeds in a hot, dry pan until golden. Remove and set aside.

- Heat the avocado oil in a large wok or frying pan and add the mushrooms, cooking until caramelised. Add the steak slices and the marinade and fry for 2-3 minutes, adding the kale towards the end, stirring into the mixture to gently wilt.
- Add in the sesame oil and salt and pepper to taste.
- Serve over cooked cauliflower rice if desired, and top with toasted sesame seeds.

Nutritional Values per serving:

- Calories: 675 Kcal
- Sugar: 2g
- Fat: 53g
- Carbohydrates: 9g
- Fiber: 3g
- Protein: 38g

13. Keto Turkey and Vegetable Skillet

Prep Time: 10 Minutes
Cook Time: 15 Minutes
Total Time: 25 Minutes
Servings: 2

Ingredients:

- 3 tablespoons of coconut oil (90 ml), to cook with

- 0.75 lb of turkey breasts (335 g), diced (or ground turkey)
- 4 slices of bacon (112 g), diced
- 1/2 medium onion (55 g), diced
- 3 spears of asparagus (45 g), chopped
- 1 cup of spinach (30 g), chopped
- 4 teaspoons of fresh thyme (4 g), chopped
- Salt and pepper, to taste

Instructions:

- In a large skillet, melt the coconut oil over medium-high heat. Add the turkey and bacon to the skillet and sauté until slightly browned about 5 to 7 minutes.
- Add the onion, asparagus, spinach and fresh thyme to the skillet. Sauté for an additional 10 minutes until the turkey and bacon are cooked through and the vegetables are soft.
- Season with salt and pepper, to taste.

Nutritional Values per serving:

- Calories: 665 Kcal
- Sugar: 2g
- Fat: 52g
- Carbohydrates: 5g
- Fiber: 2g

- Protein: 47g

14. Vegan thai soup

Prep time: 10 Minutes

Cook time: 15 Minutes

Total time: 25 Minutes

Servings: 3-4

You only need one pot to make this delicious vegan Thai soup. It's made with easy to get ingredients and you can add your favorite veggies.

Ingredients:

- 1/2 julienned red onion
- 1/2 julienned red bell pepper
- 3 sliced mushrooms
- 2 cloves of garlic, finely chopped
- 1/2-inch piece of ginger root (about 1 cm), peeled and finely chopped
- 1/2 Thai chili, finely chopped*
- 2 cups vegetable broth or water (500 ml)
- 1 14-ounce can coconut milk (400 ml)
- 1 tbsp coconut, cane or brown sugar
- 10 oz firm tofu, cubed (275 g)
- 1 tbsp tamari or soy sauce
- The juice of half a lime

- A handful of fresh cilantro, chopped

Instructions:

- Place all the veggies (onion, red bell pepper, mushrooms, garlic, ginger and Thai chili), broth, coconut milk and sugar in a large pot.
- Bring it to a boil and then cook over medium heat for about 5 minutes.
- Add the tofu and cook for 5 minutes more.
- Remove from the heat, add the tamari, lime juice and fresh cilantro. Stir and serve.
- Keep the soup in a sealed container in the fridge for up to 5 days. You can also freeze it.

Notes:

* Feel free to use any type of chili you want.

Nutritional Values per serving:

- Calories: 339 Kcal
- Sugar: 5.3g
- Fat: 27.6g
- Carbohydrates: 15.6g
- Fiber: 3.2g
- Protein: 14.8g

15. Vegan Cauliflower Fried Rice

Prep Time: 10 Minutes

Cook Time :15 Minutes

Total Time :25 Minutes

Servings: 3

Ingredients:

- 1/2 tsp oil (optional)
- 1/4 cup (40 g) onion or shallots, chopped
- 4 cloves of garlic finely chopped
- 1 tbsp minced ginger
- 1 cup (140 g) peas and carrots
- 1/2 cup (74.5 g) chopped bell pepper
- 1/2 (0.5) head of medium cauliflower, 2.5 to 3 cups shredded
- 1/4 (0.25) head of broccoli, about 1 cup shredded, or use more cauliflower
- 1 tbsp + 1 tsp soy sauce
- 1 to 2 tsp sambal oelek or asian chile sauce
- 1/2 to 1 tsp toasted sesame oil
- 1/4 tsp (0.25 tsp) salt
- A generous dash of black pepper
- Scallions for garnish

Instructions:

- Cook onion and garlic in oil (or 1 tbsp broth) over medium heat until golden. Add ginger, bell pepper, veggies, peas and carrots and a dash of salt. Mix, cover and cook for 3 to 4 minutes.

- Add the shredded cauliflower or cauliflower+ broccoli, sauces, salt and pepper and mix well.

- Cover and cook for 5 minutes. Fluff really well, cover and let sit to steam for another 2 minutes. You want the cauliflower to be cooked to a bit more than al dente, but still have just a slight bite.

- Taste and adjust salt, flavor. Fluff again. Serve hot as is or with some stir fry or baked tofu. Add some asian chile sauce or some soy sauce for garnish when serving as is. You can serve it with some stir fry like the Baked Tofu and Eggplant with Soy Lime Sauce.

Notes:

To add egg sub: Crumble up 1/4 cup tofu and add to the pan at step 1 after the onions have cooked. Cook until heated through, add a good pinch of turmeric and Indian black salt (kala namak) and mix. Continue adding the ginger and veggies.

Add some toasted nuts with the cauliflower for variation.

Use coconut aminos to make soy-free.

Nutritional Values per serving:

- Calories: 106 Kcal
- Fat: 3g
- Carbohydrates: 17g
- Fiber: 5g
- Protein: 5g

16. Easy Keto Chili

Prep time: 10 Minutes

Cook time: 30 Minutes

Total time: 40 Minutes

Servings: 6

Ingredients:

- 1 pound of lean ground beef
- 2 cloves garlic crushed
- 1 tablespoon olive oil
- 1 medium onion roughly chopped
- 28 oz can crushed tomato
- 1 cup of chopped cherry tomatoes
- 1 cup of water
- 1 ½ teaspoons of sea salt
- 2 tablespoons of chili powder
- ½ tsp ground cayenne pepper
- 1 tablespoon of cumin powder
- 1 teaspoon of garlic powder

- 2 teaspoons of onion powder

Instructions:

- Brown the ground beef, onions, garlic
- Add the can of tomatoes, fresh tomatoes, water, and spices.
- Allow to simmer on medium low heat for 30-45 minutes.
- Alternatively you can cook this chili in slow cooker to do so refer to the notes section.
- This recipe double and freezes well.

Recipe Notes:

Slow Cooker Instructions:

- Add all the ingredients into your slow cooker and break up the ground beef and then set to low. Your Keto Chili will be done in 4-6 hours, based on your specific slow cooker.

Nutritional Values per serving:

- Calories: 178 Kcal
- Fat: 5.5g
- Carbohtydrates: 7.3g
- Fiber: 2.2g
- Sugar: 2.2g

- Protein: 24.3g

17. Keto Air Fryer Fish Sticks

Prep Time: 10 Minutes

Cook Time: 10 Minutes

Total Time: 20 Minutes

Servings: 4

Ingredients:

- 1 lb white fish such as cod
- 1/4 cup mayonnaise
- 2 tbsp Dijon mustard
- 2 tbsp water
- 1 1/2 cups pork rind panko such as Pork King Good
- 3/4 tsp cajun seasoning
- Salt and pepper to taste

Instructions:

- Spray the air fryer rack with non-stick cooking spray (I use avocado oil spray).
- Pat the fish dry and cut into sticks about 1 inch by 2 inches wide (how you are able to cut it will depend a little on what kind of fish you buy and how thick and wide it is).

- In a small shallow bowl, whisk together the mayo, mustard, and water. In another shallow bowl, whisk together the pork rinds and Cajun seasoning. Add salt and pepper to taste (both the pork rinds and seasoning could have a fair bit of salt, so dip a finger in to taste how salty it is).
- Working with one piece of fish at a time, dip into the mayo mixture to coat and then tap off the excess. Dip into the pork rind mixture and toss to coat. Place on the air fryer rack.
- Set to Air Fry at 400F and bake 5 minutes, the flip the fish sticks with tongs and bake another 5 minutes. Serve immediately.

Recipe Notes:

If you don't have an air fryer, you can still make these delicious keto fish sticks. Simply preheat your oven to 425F and add several tablespoons of oil to a rimmed sheet pan. Place the sheet pan in the oven while it preheats. Place the coated fish sticks on the pan and bake 5 minutes, then flip over and bake another 5 minutes.

Nutritional Values per serving :

- Fat: 16g
- Carbohydrates: 1g
- Fiber: 0.5g

- Protein: 26.4g
- Calories: 263 kcal

18. Keto zuppa toscana

Prep Time: 10 Minutes

Cook Time: 45 Minutes

Total Time: 55 Minutes

Servings: 8

Ingredients:

- 6 slices bacon, roughly chopped
- 1 lb ground mild Italian sausage
- 1 tbsp (14g) butter
- 2 tsp (10g) minced garlic
- ½ tsp ground sage
- ¼ tsp black pepper
- 2 ¾ cups chicken broth
- ¾ cup heavy whipping cream
- ¼ cup shredded parmesan cheese
- 1 lb radishes, quartered
- 2 oz kale, de-stemmed, roughly chopped

Instructions:

- To a large pot over medium heat, cook chopped bacon until crisp. Transfer bacon to a paper-towel-lined plate and dispose of grease, but do not wash the pan.

- In the same pot over medium-high heat, cook ground sausage until browned, breaking the meat apart with a wooden spoon while cooking. Transfer browned sausage to a paper towel-lined plate and dispose of grease, but do not wash the pan.

- To same pot over medium heat, melt butter. Add garlic and spices and sauté until fragrant, about 1 minute. Increase heat to medium-high and add in chicken broth, heavy cream, and shredded parmesan. Bring mixture to a simmer, add quartered radishes, and decrease the heat to medium-low. Simmer until radishes are fork-tender, about 15-20 minutes.

- Stir in browned sausage and chopped kale and continue to simmer until kale wilts, about 5-10 minutes, before serving in bowls. Garnish soup with crisped bacon crumbles.

Nutritional Values per serving:

- Calories: 334 Kcal
- Fat: 31g
- Carbohydrates: 3.9g
- Dietary Fiber: 1.1g
- Protein: 12g

19. Taco Casseroele - Low Carb/Keto

Prep time: 20 Minutes

Cook time: 20 Minutes

Total time: 40 Minutes

Servings: 6

Ingredients:

- 1 1/2 lb ground beef
- 1 14.5 oz can chopped tomatoes
- 1 4 oz can diced green chiles
- 2 cups cooked cauliflower rice
- 3 tbs taco seasoning
- 1 8 oz bag taco cheese

Instructions:

- Cook the cauliflower rice (either bagged or fresh) and pat dry to remove excess moisture.
- Cook beef on stovetop until brown.
- Add tomatoes, cauliflower, taco seasoning and chiles and stir until well mixed.
- In a 13 x 9 baking dish, layer enough of the beef mixture to cover the bottom - about half.
- Top with 2/3 of the cheese and spread evenly.
- Repeat with the rest of the beef and then top with the rest of the cheese.

- Bake for 15-20 min at 350 degrees until cheese is melted.
- Serve in a bowl alone or with sour cream and avocado.

Nutritional Values per serving:

- Calories: 522 Kcal
- Fat: 31g
- Carbohydrates: 10g
- Fiber: 3g
- Protein: 42g

20. Broccoli Bacon Salad with Onions and Coconut Cream

Prep Time: 10 Minutes

Cook Time: 30 Minutes

Total Time: 40 Minutes

Servings: 6

Ingredients:

- 1 lb broccoli florets
- 4 small red onions or 2 large ones, sliced
- 20 slices of bacon, chopped into small pieces
- 1 cup coconut cream
- Salt to taste

Instructions:

- Cook the bacon first, and then cook the onions in the bacon fat.
- Blanche the broccoli florets (or you can use them raw or have them softer by boiling them).
- Toss the bacon pieces, onions, and broccoli florets together with the coconut cream and salt to taste.
- Serve at room temperature.

Nutritional Values per serving:

Serving Size: 1 bowl

- Calories: 280 Kcal
- Sugar: 2g
- Fat: 26g
- Carbohydrates: 8g
- Fiber: 3g
- Protein: 7g

21. Keto Chicken Mushroom Casserole

Prep Time: 10 Minutes
Cook Time: 40 Minutes
Total Time: 50 Minutes
Servings: 4

Ingredients:

- 4 tablespoons of avocado oil (30 ml), to cook with

- 8 chicken thighs (with skin on) (1.2 kg)
- 1 medium onion (110 g), peeled and thinly sliced
- 3 cloves of garlic (9 g), peeled and chopped
- 2 tablespoons of fresh rosemary (6 g), chopped
- 30 white button mushrooms (300 g), halved
- 2 oz of kale (56 g)
- Salt and freshly ground black pepper
- Additional rosemary sprigs for garnish (optional)

Instructions:

- Preheat the oven to 350°F (180°C).
- Add avocado oil to a frying pan and brown the chicken thighs skin-side down until golden and crispy, then turn the thighs over and cook the other side for a minute or two.
- The chicken isn't cooked right now, but will be finished off in the oven. Carefully remove from the frying pan and put into a roasting dish.
- Using the leftover oil in the pan, cook the sliced onions, garlic and rosemary and cook over a low-moderate heat to soften the onions completely. Turn the heat up and keep cooking the onions for a few more minutes until they become jammy. Add the mushrooms to the frying pan for a few minutes.

- Spoon the mushrooms and jammy onions into the roasting tray around the chicken pieces and place the dish in the oven for 20 minutes.
- In the meantime, toss the kale in some more olive oil.
- After 20 minutes, increase the oven temperature to 400 F (200 C) and remove the tray from the oven while it heats. Scatter the oiled kale in and around the dish, then return the dish to the oven for an additional 5 minutes.
- Season with salt and freshly ground black pepper, as well as additional rosemary sprigs, then serve to the table for everyone to help themselves.

Nutritional Values per serving:

- Calories: 553 Kcal
- Sugar: 3g
- Fat: 42g
- Carbohydrates: 7g
- Fiber: 2g
- Protein: 35g

22. 3-Ingredient Creamy Keto Salmon "Pasta" Recipe

Prep Time: 5 Minutes

Cook Time: 5 Minutes

Total Time: 10 Minutes

Servings: 2

Ingredients:

- 2 tablespoons of coconut oil (30 ml), to cook with
- 8 oz of smoked salmon (224 g), diced
- 2 zucchinis (240 g), spiraled or use a peeler to make into long noodle-like strands
- 1/4 cup of mayo (60 ml)

Instructions:

- In a skillet, melt the coconut oil over medium-high heat. Add the smoked salmon and sauté until slightly browned, about 2 to 3 minutes.
- Add the zucchini "noodles" to the skillet and sauté until soft, about 1 to 2 minutes.
- Add the mayo to the skillet, stirring well to combine.
- Divide the "pasta" between 2 plates and serve.

Nutritional Values per serving:

- Calories: 470 Kcal
- Sugar: 2g
- Fat: 42g
- Carbohydrates: 4g
- Fiber: 1g
- Protein: 21g

23. Mini Spinach Meatloaves

Prep Time: 5 Minutes

Cook Time: 20 Minutes

Total Time: 25 Minutes

Yield: 12 Muffins

Ingredients:

- 1/4 lb (113 g) ground pork or ground turkey
- 1/4 lb(113 g) ground beef
- 1/2 small onion (55 g), diced
- 2 cloves garlic, minced
- 1/3 lb (140 g) fresh spinach, chopped small
- 4 eggs, whisked
- 2 tablespoons Italian seasoning
- 1/2 tablespoon salt
- 1/2 teaspoon black pepper
- 1/3 cup (80 ml) almond or coconut milk
- Coconut oil to sauté in

Instructions:

- Preheat oven to 400 F (200 C).
- Saute the meat, diced onions, and garlic in 1 tablespoon of coconut oil. When the meat is cooked, add in the chopped spinach and sauté for 1-2 minutes longer.
- Place muffin cup liners into a 12-cup muffin pan.

- In a large bowl, combine the sauté with the whisked eggs, Italian seasoning, salt, black pepper, and almond or coconut milk.
- Divide the mixture between the 12 muffin cups.
- Bake for 10 minutes until each muffin is pretty solid. Cook for longer if the muffins are still liquidy.

Nutritional Values per serving:

Serving Size: 6 muffins

- Calories: 430 Kcal
- Sugar: 2g
- Fat: 30g
- Carbohydrates: 7g
- Fiber: 3g
- Protein: 30g

24. Cobb Egg Salad

Prep Time: 15 Minutes
Cook Time: 10 Minutes
Total Time: 25 Minutes
Servings: 4

Ingredients:

- 3 tablespoons nonfat plain yogurt
- 3 tablespoons low-fat mayonnaise

- ¼ teaspoon garlic powder
- ¼ teaspoon freshly ground pepper
- ⅛ teaspoon salt
- 8 hard-boiled eggs (see Tip)
- 1 ripe avocado, cubed
- 2 slices bacon, cooked and crumbled
- ¼ cup crumbled blue cheese

Instructions:

- Combine yogurt, mayonnaise, garlic powder, pepper and salt in a medium bowl.
- Halve eggs and discard 4 of the yolks (or save for another use).
- Add whites and the remaining 4 yolks to the bowl and mash to desired consistency.
- Gently stir in avocado, bacon and blue cheese.

Make Ahead Tip: Cover and refrigerate for up to 2 days.

Tip: To hard-boil eggs, place eggs in a single layer in a saucepan; cover with water. Bring to a simmer over medium-high heat. Reduce heat to low and cook at the barest simmer for 10 minutes. Remove from heat, pour out hot water and cover the eggs with ice-cold water. Let stand until cool enough to handle before peeling.

Nutritional Values per serving:

- Serving size: about ¾ cup
- Calories: 235 Kcal
- Fat: 17g
- Fiber: 3g
- Carbohydrates: 9g
- Protein: 3g

CONCLUSION

Intermittent fasting isn't starving yourself to lose weight right. Intermittent fasting isn't a diet. It's a pattern of eating. To be more exact, it's a lifestyle to carry on for life.

And as a lifestyle, it's very important to track and measure your progress.

In conclusion, intermittent fasting is one of the simplest and most effective methods you have to improve your overall wellbeing and is a great tool for weight management.

Did you enjoy this book? I will be very pleased if you leave a review on Amazon, and also share your thoughts with me.

Made in the
USA
Monee, IL